MEMOIR
OF A LIVING
DISEASE

MAURICE MIERAU

MEMOIR
OF A LIVING
DISEASE

THE STORY OF EARL HERSHFIELD AND
TUBERCULOSIS
IN MANITOBA AND BEYOND

GREAT PLAINS
PUBLICATIONS

Great Plains Publications
420 – 70 Arthur Street
Winnipeg, MB R3B 1G7
www.greatplains.mb.ca

Great Plains Publications gratefully acknowledges the financial support provided for its publishing program by the Government of Canada through the Book Publishing Industry Development Program (BPIDP); the Canada Council for the Arts; as well as the Manitoba Department of Culture, Heritage and Tourism; and the Manitoba Arts Council.

Design & Typography by Relish Design Studio Inc.
Printed in Canada by Friesens

CANADIAN CATALOGUING IN PUBLICATION DATA

LIBRARY AND ARCHIVES CANADA CATALOGUING IN PUBLICATION

Main entry under title:

Mierau, Maurice, 1962-
    Memoir of a living disease : the story of Earl Hershfield
and tuberculosis in Manitoba and beyond / Maurice Mierau.

ISBN 1-894283-49-X

    1. Tuberculosis--Manitoba. 2. Hershfield, Earl S., 1934-.
I. Title.

RA644.T7M44 2004   614.5'42'097127   C2004-904009-X

Dedicated to the memory of Carl Ridd, 1929-2003,
who believed you can change things with words.

ACKNOWLEDGEMENTS

While writing this book I have acquired more debts than I can repay or adequately acknowledge here. I want to thank the Manitoba Lung Association and the late John Hutchings, their executive director, for trusting me to write this book and for providing financial support. Thanks as well to Dr. Peter Warren, who read the manuscript on behalf of the Manitoba Lung Association, and to Earl Hershfield for spending many hours talking to me and reviewing the manuscript. My gratitude goes to my wife, Betsy Troutt, who provided crucial feedback on an early draft, and put up with me when things weren't going well. Any errors in this book are entirely my own.

Thanks to the wonderful staff at Great Plains for all their work.

I want to acknowledge the following people for granting me interviews and helping me understand tuberculosis, public health, history, and the many other things we talked about:

Nick Anthonisen, Alan Artibise, Ron Birt, Kym Blackwood, Reuben Cherniack, George Comstock, Hubert Drouin, Lawrence Elliott, Kevin Elwood, Donald Enarson, Anne Fanning, Margaret Fast, Sharon Fletcher, Phil Fontaine, Patrick Friesen, Kim Froese, Brian Gushulak, Gordon Guyatt, James Hanley, Al Harmacy, Beth Henning, Philip Hopewell, Michael Iseman, Jay Johnson, Arlene Jones, Wayne Kepron, Jay Keystone, Joann MacMorran, Robert Marks, Evelyn McGarrol, Alfred Monnin, Arnold Naimark, Rick O'Brien, Gwynne Oosterbaan, Pam Orr, Rey Pagtakhan, David Penman, David Peters, Frank Plummer, Michael Rattray, Lee Reichman, Judy Riedel, Marion Roth, Ann Russell, John Sbarbaro, David B. Stewart, Peter Warren, Nancy Williamson, Joyce Wolfe, Jim Zayshley and Lynn Jaworski.

Many thanks to Phil Fontaine, Joann MacMorran, Merrell-Ann Pharc, and Andrew Troutt, for various kinds of indispensable assistance.

Thanks are due as well to Frank Hechter and Joy Letkemann of the Manitoba Lung Association, and to the staff at the Provincial Archives of Manitoba and the Western Canada Pictorial Index.

A number of my informants and interview subjects did not want to be named, but their input was nonetheless important. Apologies to anyone I have inadvertently failed to acknowledge.

TABLE OF CONTENTS

PROLOGUE

"INTEREST IN TUBERCULOSIS IS AT AN ALL-TIME LOW WHICH
IS CERTAINLY STRIKING [SINCE] DEATHS ARE AT AN ALL-TIME HIGH."
— DR. PAUL FARMER, *INFECTIONS AND INEQUALITIES: THE MODERN PLAGUES*

It is a cold day in the winter of 1986 in downtown Winnipeg. A short man in a tweed jacket, carrying a black doctor's bag, hurries into the skywalk between the Somerset building and Eaton's. He walks up to two men who stand with their backs against the glass of the skywalk, paying no attention to the rush hour traffic flowing below. The men look like Laurel and Hardy, one tall, the other short, both hatless. Neither man has shaved recently and their clothes are rumpled, probably doubling as bedclothes. Over the last few minutes they've been sidling up to passersby and asking, respectfully but in a mumble, if they can have some change. Mostly they get nothing. Both of them smell faintly of alcohol.

The man in the tweed jacket greets the panhandlers by name. He jokes about the weather, moving quickly all the time, and they grin back at him. They each take a paper cup with four large pills in it, swallow the pills one at a time, and drink some water. After they finish taking the pills their visitor records something on a clipboard and then packs up his doctor's bag. He leaves them with a brusque goodbye, although his patients wouldn't call it that if anybody asked them, and descends through the Somerset Building to find his Toyota on the frozen Winnipeg streets.

Seventeen years later, the end of 2003. The same man, in the same tweed jacket with a white lab coat thrown over it, enters an isolation room in Ward H6 of Winnipeg's respiratory hospital. There's a young woman lying there. She looks anorexic, her arm protruding from the sheets like a barely-covered bone. Her mother is sitting beside the bed, and she asks the man why, after taking 12 pills a day for a week, her daughter is not feeling better. He says it will take a few weeks before she feels better, and the mother seems resigned to that.

The man goes to his office, where a nurse is interviewing an Aboriginal man whose girlfriend was just admitted to the hospital. She is comatose with TB at the age of 29 and she will probably die. Her only addresses were the Main Street Project, a shelter for homeless people, and the Colony Soup Kitchen. Her chest x-rays are in the basement, and the man in the lab coat goes down to look at them. They show a white haze over her lungs that looks like cotton candy punctuated with black holes. These holes are the cavities where the disease eats away the lung's ability to breathe, gradually choking her. After viewing her x-rays, the man walks briskly out to his Toyota in the hospital parking lot.

The man's name is Dr. Earl Hershfield. For Earl these were just regular days at the office, working to control a disease that most Canadians assume went away at some time in the hazy, distant past. This is the story of a disease that won't go away, and also an account of Earl's lifelong effort to make that story end.

Imagine a disease that is the most successful mass-murderer currently alive on earth, killing at least two million people every year. That works out to one human being dead every fifteen seconds. This is a disease that kills about 300,000 children per year, according to the World Health Organization. Now imagine that this same disease is entirely preventable and curable and has been since the 1960s. Imagine that the World Bank, 12 years ago, announced that of all the infectious diseases, this one was the most cost-effective to treat. Why are we still watching millions of people die of tuberculosis, never mind writing books about it?

Tuberculosis, or TB, is an infectious disease caused by a germ called the tubercle bacillus. The tubercle bacillus was discovered by Robert Koch in 1882 and is still raging out of control worldwide. Tuberculosis spreads through the air, so if someone is infectious they infect others simply by coughing or sneezing. You don't need a mosquito or polluted water or body fluid exchange to spread TB, although any of those things might help weaken your immune system. You just need to breathe in enough TB germs from someone who is infectious. "Ebola with wings" is how Richard Bumgarner of the World Health Organization described TB in 1993.

People who are poor, don't have jobs or decent houses, don't have enough to eat (like many people with AIDS) are more vulnerable to TB than anyone else. Doctors call these people *immuno-compromised*. TB and AIDS are the two biggest killers in the world, especially in combination. HIV/AIDS kills the immune system, but something else has to come along to kill the immuno-compromised individual. That something else, more than anything, is TB. The average survival time for the millions who have both advanced AIDS and active TB is five weeks. The AIDS epidemic in Africa cannot be stopped without stopping TB.

Oddly, not everyone who is infected with the germ gets sick with the disease. What is the distinction between getting infected with TB, called having latent TB, and getting sick with it? This is maybe the strangest thing about tuberculosis. You can get infected without getting sick. If you breathe in the tubercle bacillus there is a very good chance that your immune system successfully fights it off. You will test positive on a skin test for TB, but you aren't sick — for the time being. However, 10% of the people who get infected become actively ill with TB within two years of exposure. Globally, about 3 billion people every year become infected with TB. In them the disease is latent, a deadly lurker.

Why do only 10% of those infected with TB develop an active case of the disease? Why do a handful of people develop the disease decades after exposure? Earl Hershfield says that if you can answer those questions definitively you are guaranteed a Nobel Prize in medicine. One community health nurse says, "it's a weird disease." Precisely because of TB's weirdness it is difficult to control and sometimes very hard to treat.

So the answer to the question of why those of us in the wealthy countries of the G-8 have allowed the world tuberculosis epidemic to flourish is a combination of science, history, and politics. The simplest answer, though, is that the disease is invisible to the citizens of countries in the wealthy northern hemisphere of the globe. An overwhelming 99% of the deaths from tuberculosis worldwide happen in the world's poorest countries. And that doesn't count many of the AIDS patients who actually died of TB. Every year international health organizations, desperate to get funding, fight about whether deaths should go in the AIDS column or the TB column. Here in Canada, complacency is almost logical; we get the disease at a rate of only 5.5 people per 100,000. In the late 1960s, when Earl Hershfield's career began, the rate was about 30 per 100,000. But the Canadians that TB affects today are primarily Aboriginal people and first-generation immigrants, who are often marginalized in Canadian society, and who get the disease at the high rates that persist in the developing world. Because TB has become invisible to most Canadians, it is no wonder that our public health officials have trouble getting money from politicians obsessed with lowering taxes.

TB matters now because public health is a global security issue, and we are facing a global TB epidemic. People who are chronically sick and desperately poor make good terrorists: they have nothing to lose. That's why public health is more effective in the war on terrorism than an Abrams tank. But along with arms, the G-8 countries have exported the human misery that accompanied the original Industrial Revolution. Public health has always eroded along with explosions of poverty, both in the country and the city. If nothing else, we have become very good at counting the economic and human cost of the devastation that TB brings. The global invoice for our astonishing neglect of TB is US $12 billion per year in lost productivity alone. Less than 50% of the TB cases worldwide are diagnosed and of those only 60% are actually cured. If the current trends continue, by the year 2020 some 200 million people will get TB and 36 million of them will die. Calling this an epidemic seems like an understatement.

TB cases in Canada have been rising since 1989 as part of a global resurgence of the disease that started in the late 1980s and then snowballed through the 1990s, with no sign of abatement yet. While there were only 124 cases in Manitoba for 2003, which sounds like a small number, that's almost a 25% increase over the previous year. In addition, the disease has a disproportionate effect on two groups: Aboriginal people and immigrants and refugees from countries where there's a lot of TB. Almost half the active cases of TB in Manitoba for 2002 were Aboriginal people, and almost a third were among the "foreign born". There is an outbreak of the disease on a First Nations community in Manitoba almost every year. Often particular Aboriginal reserves have repeated outbreaks. There is no great mystery in this — unemployment, overcrowded housing, substance abuse, malnutrition and despair are powerful blows to the human immune system.

As for immigrants and refugees, they come from Asia, Africa, the Caribbean, and Latin America, all places where TB is still a common disease. A map that displayed income and TB levels would show a simple inverse relationship: low income and poor public health infrastructure is accompanied by high prevalence of TB. India, China, sub-Saharan Africa, Vietnam, Ethiopia, the Philippines, Russia, all have high rates of the disease. 80% of all the TB patients in the world live in the 22 countries with the highest incidence of the disease. The fact is that poor people reproduce faster than rich ones do too, so their case numbers increase more quickly while their resources stretch even thinner.

While TB is an excluded disease for those applying for immigration to Canada, meaning that Canadian immigrants cannot have active TB, that doesn't stop people with latent disease from being admitted. These immigrants need treatment after they arrive in Canada because of infections they got in their country of origin. Within the first few years of arriving, they tend to get sick with TB at about the same rate they would at home. And sometimes refugees come into Canada who need treatment for TB, as with the Chilean refugees in the 1970s, the Vietnamese in the 1980s, and the Sudanese right now. The world keeps producing more refugees too: they have increased at a nine-fold rate over the last 20 years, and the World Health Organization estimates that 50% of them are infected with TB.

Most immigrants to Canada settle in Ontario, British Columbia, Alberta, and Quebec, and this population tends to get most of the TB. Manitoba, Saskatchewan, and northern Canada are different: they get fewer immigrants but have proportionately more Aboriginal people. And it is these communities, both on and off reserve, who suffer the most with TB. To make matters worse, diabetes is one of the biggest risk factors for getting TB, and Aboriginal people get diabetes at an unusually high rate. Most Canadians rarely see or think about this epidemic of suffering and loss. After all, the numbers aren't very big, and many of the people who get TB live far from the city while some of the unhealthiest live under bridges and in shelters for the homeless. No matter how good our intentions, out of sight really does mean out of mind. And the ugly spectre of racism hovers over the scene, blotting good intentions and reminding us that the indigenous people of Canada are also the poorest and sickest among us.

I wrote this book as a memoir of a living disease, and also the account of one man's outstanding career in public health, fighting that same disease. I tell the story of the Ninette Sanatorium and the origins of the Manitoba Lung Association, and also the story of TB treatment in an international context. There is commentary by nurses and doctors who work with the disease here in Manitoba, and also by internationally recognized experts on TB, many of whom are Earl Hershfield's colleagues and friends. I tell the story of some of the communities who struggle with TB, including the story of outbreaks that continue to affect inner city Winnipeg and an isolated northern community. The book concludes with an account of Earl's international career and a chapter on the future of a disease that really ought to be dead.

Earl Hershfield's career is a reminder that Manitobans and Canadians can make a difference in the world. It is also a reminder that, while a lot of money has been spent on TB research and control in the last few years, much work still needs to be done. You cannot have good public health in a world where so many people are staggeringly poor, and doctors alone can never solve this problem. In the end if we cannot heal our own indifference to the suffering of others, we will get exactly the kind of world we deserve. Earl Hershfield's career has been a struggle not just against tuberculosis, but also against the indifference of the affluent.

1

STARTING A CAREER

The Sanatorium Board of Manitoba, from 1904 through to the 1960s, did what its name implied: it operated specialized hospitals called sanatoria for the treatment of tuberculosis. This form of institutional care was in fact the international standard for treating TB through the first half of the 20th century. TB patients were secluded in a sanatorium or a TB hospital. Before the advent of effective drug treatment in the 1960s, sanatorium treatment consisted of "rest therapy," or bed rest, improved nutrition, and various forms of lung surgery. When TB drugs started to empty sanatorium beds, and long before it became fashionable to talk about doing community-based health care, the Sanatorium Board was faced with a daunting challenge. They needed to get out of the sanatorium business, develop a new kind of TB control program, and most importantly find new talent to run the program. What they didn't know yet was they needed Earl Hershfield.

In 1963 Earl Hershfield had just finished his medical studies at the Mayo Clinic in Rochester, Minnesota, and moved back home with his family to Winnipeg. Earl went into practice with his father Sheppy and his uncle Harry at 294 Portage Avenue in what was then called the Somerset Building. Earl enjoyed working with his family, but he did not enjoy family medicine. He wanted to be a specialist, to use his training as a chest physician. Instead he spent mornings visiting hospitals and making himself visible so that he would get consultations, and then spent afternoons in the office seeing patients. He was restless.

Earl was already interested in TB from his medical education, so in 1964 he went to see Dr. Tony (D.L.) Scott, who had been running the Sanatorium Board's Central Tuberculosis Clinic in Winnipeg for 34 years. Scott hired Earl as a medical consultant, and so in 1964 Earl started working for the Sanatorium Board on a half-time basis. Over the next three years Earl says "I really learned about TB, how to read chest x-rays, and what to do about the results of chest x-rays." And it turned out that what Earl wanted to do was exactly what the Sanatorium Board needed – modern TB treatment.

By the late 1960s the Sanatorium Board of Manitoba was facing major change. The introduction of effective drug treatment for tuberculosis meant that the disease was now nearly always curable, and also that sanatoria were fast becoming obsolete. At its peak, the Sanatorium Board operated a large sanatorium at Ninette, and much smaller facilities at Brandon, Clearwater Lake, Dynevor, and the Central Tuberculosis Clinic in Winnipeg. The sanatoria other than Ninette all housed Aboriginal and Inuit patients, and the Clinic mostly served as an outpatient facility – there were only 30 beds and longer term patients were usually sent to Ninette. Successful drug treatment emptied these institutions all over the province and indeed the world, making them expensive and unnecessary, but also leaving a vacuum. In Manitoba the doctors who had run the TB sanatoria were all approaching retirement age. Medical schools were no longer producing TB doctors, and the remaining sanatoria couldn't afford to hire the modern lung disease specialists coming onto the job market.

In retrospect, Earl's emerging interest in TB was well-timed. But TB treatment was not generally attracting ambitious young doctors in the 1960s, partly because the period was marked by capacity reductions and sanatorium closures. Governments were not interested in funding specialized institutions full of empty beds. In Manitoba, the sanatoria at Clearwater Lake and Brandon were converted to chronic care facilities because of lessening demand for TB beds. Then in 1965, Clearwater Lake was closed down completely, and in the same year the Sanatorium Board turned over Assiniboine Hospital, formerly the Brandon Sanatorium, to the province.

OBSTACLES

The Sanatorium Board was going to have to transform itself from a body that administered TB facilities into a community health organization, but before doing that there was an obstacle. It would have to deal with closing down the largest and best-known sanatorium in the province, Manitoba Sanatorium, located on the shores of Pelican Lake just outside Ninette. The institution had opened in 1910, and touched the lives of thousands of Manitobans over the next 62 years. It was the major employer in the town of Ninette, and the major enterprise of the Sanatorium Board. In this pre-medicare era, the Ninette sanatorium was built with government money and also money raised through Christmas Seals campaigns over many years. At its peak it had 400 beds, 24 buildings, and 90 employees. Closing this institution would prove painful.

Robert Marks was the Board's financial controller from 1959 until 1973 and also their executive director from 1981 to 1994. He says that the writing was on the wall for the Ninette sanatorium by 1967:

The patient population at Ninette kept going down through the late 1960s. You had about 70 people rattling around and a bed capacity of about 400. The provincial government was forking out the money, but questions were beginning to be asked. And the Board itself could see the end in sight. Now that was easier said than done because the roots of institutional care ran pretty deep, not within administration, but within one aspect of the medical administration.

What Marks alludes to here is that there would be no change until the key medical personnel retired. Dr. Eddy (E.L.) Ross retired in 1967 as Medical Director of the Sanatorium Board after 40 years in the position. Dr. Tony Scott retired in 1969 as director of the Central Tuberculosis Clinic in Winnipeg. And Dr. A.L. Paine, who was the last medical director at Ninette, retired in 1972. The stage was now set for the last and most difficult change. Marks says that "as long as Ross, Scott, and Paine were in the picture, it was institutional care, the status quo, but you could pretty well see that wasn't going to work anymore."

A NEW VISION

Earl Hershfield describes Jack (T.A.J.) Cunnings as a visionary because of the way in which he re-structured and modernized the Sanatorium Board of Manitoba in the 1960s. Jack Cunnings, like many early administrators and healthcare workers in TB, was an ex-patient. He got TB in 1937 and was admitted to the Ninette San. As a banker, and an energetic personality, he quickly became bored with the regimen of constant rest at the San. After he recovered, Cunnings pushed for more job training for people in long term sanatorium care, and eventually became Rehabilitation Director at the Central Tuberculosis Clinic in Winnipeg. By 1945 he was Secretary-Treasurer of the Board. Ironically it was Jack Cunnings who would preside, as executive director of the Sanatorium Board, over the eventual demise of the Ninette San.

As executive director of the San Board, Cunnings was one of the driving forces behind building Winnipeg's Rehabilitation Hospital on Sherbrook Street, which opened in 1962 (it is now part of the Health Sciences Centre). The Rehab Hospital worked with people recovering from respiratory diseases like TB, and with TB numbers going down, it was a way for the San Board to move into a new area. It was the first specialized rehabilitation hospital in Canada. The new building also became the home of the Central Tuberculosis Clinic in early 1962, and the clinic's name was changed to the D.A. Stewart Centre for Respiratory Disease in 1968. The name change was significant in that it symbolized a shift away from an exclusive focus on TB.

By the late 1960s Cunnings had set the Sanatorium Board on the path to broadening its focus and surviving in a future where there would be less TB in Manitoba. But if all the sanatoria and TB hospitals were going to close, how would the remaining TB patients get treatment, and where would the medical staff be located? Given that no young TB doctors were emerging from medical schools, and that the young chest physicians commanded bigger salaries than the Sanatorium Board could afford, what was the solution? For the first time the Sanatorium Board, with Cunnings' leadership, looked at a joint venture with another institution, the University of Manitoba's Faculty of Medicine. Dr. Reuben Cherniack had already helped establish what would be a prestigious and growing respiratory disease section at the university. Cherniack, however, wanted to run the respiratory medicine program and do research – he had no desire to run a TB control program. Cunnings still needed to find a new director, but a possible structure was there: joint appointments with the university would give the Sanatorium Board access to a specialist physician who could run their flagship program.

BECOMING DIRECTOR

In late 1966 Earl got a call from Reuben Cherniack. "I was the only other young chest physician in town at the time," says Earl, and "Cherniack wanted to specialize in lung disease." They met in a hospital cafeteria, and Earl recalls Cherniack joking that "you've seen two cases of TB, I've seen one, so you know more about it than I do." What Cherniack put on the table was a job offer for Earl to be Associate Medical Director in the new Joint Respiratory Program. Earl would be responsible for running provincial TB control, and Cherniack would become Medical Director. Earl would have to create a new program for TB control that did not revolve around the sanatorium, and he'd have to learn on the job. At this point Earl also had a few job offers in the United States. One of them was in Palm Springs, California, at a one-story clinic that is now a huge multi-floor facility. Earl says, "I'd probably be a millionaire and divorced six times if I'd gone there, so I have no regrets." His Winnipeg roots and growing interest in TB made the decision easy.

So in May 1967, at the age of 33, Earl Hershfield became a full-time employee of the Sanatorium Board and the University of Manitoba, taking over Manitoba's TB control program as part of a whole series of institutional changes already underway. Appointed shortly after Earl were two other Associate Medical Directors, C.B. Schoemperlen and Louis Cherniack (Reuben's brother), also using the joint appointment model with the University of Manitoba.

MAKING THINGS CHANGE

In 1967, when Earl started his job as TB control director for Manitoba, getting TB into the mainstream of medicine was the policy of the day all over Canada and indeed all over the world. This meant the end of sanatorium treatment for the disease, the standardization and universal application of drug therapy, the end of most TB-related surgery, and also changes in case-finding, surveillance, and reporting of the disease.

Earl embraced this new era and so he had an ambitious agenda. First, he wanted to get cure rates higher by using drug therapy for all TB patients, rather than the old practice of using drugs as a supplement to a sanatorium regimen of rest and surgery. Second, he wanted to develop a control program that would administer those drugs and make sure Manitoba kept TB under control as the sanatorium era ended. Finally he wanted to see TB brought back into the mainstream of medicine, so that patients would no longer be shut away in isolated sanatoria, far from modern hospitals and often far from their families. This meant that the program would now revolve around a fully-equipped hospital and an outpatient clinic, rather than around sanatoria and TB hospitals.

Before he could implement all these changes, though, Earl needed to do a number of things to prepare the ground. He had to learn more about how to do his job, find allies for his new vision of TB control in other jurisdictions across Canada, and give nurses more responsibility for delivering care.

LEARNING ON THE JOB

In 1967 there were no textbooks, such as the one Earl would later produce with Lee Reichman, on how to run a modern tuberculosis control program. So Earl learned on the job. He tried to get his hands on everything to fully understand what was going on: he examined patients, took x-rays in the field, did tuberculin tests, administered TB vaccinations, read thousands of chest x-rays, looked at sputum samples under the microscope, and went to meetings to learn from other people who were working on TB. With no background in bacteriology, Earl even ran the tuberculosis laboratory at the Respiratory Hospital for a while. "I made my way on my own, scratching, arguing, learning, and fighting, building what many people thought was a good program," says Earl of his first five years running the program.

An important part of learning the job for Earl was traveling up north to First Nations and Inuit communities where there was a lot of TB. In 1968 Earl flew into northern Manitoba with a medical resident to take chest x-rays in a Dene community on North Knife Lake. There was no electricity there, so they brought a generator with them to operate the x-ray machine. The plane dropped them off with their equipment, and as soon as they set up the generator stopped working. The radio telephone was broken, so at this point they were stuck – the plane wouldn't be back for three days and there was nothing to do if they couldn't take x-rays.

So the resident and Earl decided to play mechanic. They tore the generator apart, and the resident, who was more mechanically inclined than Earl, thought to draw a picture and label every part as they disassembled the generator. It took over two hours to reassemble it, but the generator worked for the whole three days they were there.

But the adventure wasn't over. The return plane landed on the lake two hours late and very quickly a storm came up. The generator, x-ray camera, frame, and all the film cassettes were sitting on the dock, probably 1,000 pounds of equipment in all. It started to blow so hard that the plane was pulling away from its moorings on the finger-dock. Suddenly the finger-dock broke away from the shore. Earl tells the story:

> Here I was on the dock with heavy x-ray equipment. Fortunately – and I don't know how – I hoisted the equipment onto the plane and leaped on as the dock sunk about 100 yards from shore. This was a very cold lake, a very cold day, and who knows what would have happened. I was quite frightened.

Most of Earl's experiences were less hair-raising than this one. He recalls many pleasant meals at nursing stations in the north. Typically the visiting doctors would stay at the nursing station or in a trailer next to it since many of the communities had no motels. On one of his early visits to Eskimo Point in the Northwest Territories (now Arviat, Nunavut), he remembers being served a tasty dish of pork and rice by the nursing staff. Earl did not want to reject the meal by saying he didn't eat pork, so he discreetly pushed the pieces of meat under rice on the edges of his plate, eating his way around the pork. He thought no one noticed. But on subsequent visits to Eskimo Point and other northern communities, no one served him pork again. Word had gotten around.

"Anything I said was avant garde"

Earl Hershfield describes his first years running TB control in Manitoba like this:

> I came in there with a brashness, turning everything upside down. But I kept using data from Europe, where TB control was a high priority, and they had a long history of TB research. I continued to produce data and eventually people began to shift and then younger people got involved.

The TB control directors from the other Canadian provinces were mostly from another generation, at least 20 years older than Earl, and they were not interested in change. They did not use "much drug treatment, they were still using old methods, still had sanatoria, and so I became, at the young age of 33, the new boy on the block – anything I said was avant garde." Earl was not entirely alone. Dr. Stefan Gryzbowski was older than Earl, but he had pioneered the use of drug therapy for TB in Ontario in the 1950s, and he taught at the University of British Columbia's medical school starting in 1964. He worked extensively with

Aboriginal people and Arctic communities, and was also a consultant for international TB programs. His support for Earl was crucial in the early years of Earl's career. Dr. Anne Fanning, who teaches medicine at the University of Alberta and knew both Earl and Stefan, recalls that

> Stefan was the great godfather of tuberculosis in Canada, a wonderful Polish princely man with a brilliant mind, great passion and a wonderful sense of humour. He and Earl would debate and debate each other, and it would look like they were rivals and archenemies, but in fact they were great friends.

Gryzbowski was known, like Earl, for his iconoclasm. Dr. Don Enarson, who was Gryzbowski's student and is now an authority on TB himself, remembers his old teacher as an eccentric. Gryzbowski loved to tell ribald jokes, but only had a repertoire of six or seven. He happily repeated these in front of anyone, no matter how serious or dignified. Gryzbowski also was well-known for smoking his pipe in forbidden places, and then jamming it in a jacket pocket where it would burn a hole. He and Earl got along very well together, sharing a sense of humour and a passion for TB control.

Among the first changes that Earl Hershfield and Stefan Gryzbowski helped to inaugurate was the promotion of standard drug regimens for the treatment of TB in Canada. They also were instrumental in promoting guidelines for TB treatment, a standardized skin test, and, in 1969, a reporting system for TB. In the sanatorium era only admission statistics were kept, and so this was a major change. Now a more complete picture of patient health would be recorded on discharge from TB treatment.

Waking up the patients

In Britain, much of Europe, and the United States, the change in treating tuberculosis during the 1950s had been extremely rapid. Rest therapy, a dubious inheritance from the sanatorium era, was abandoned within five years of the introduction of effective drugs for TB. By the late 1950s the United States army was studying the effect of active exercise programs on TB patients. Having patients' bodies atrophy while their lungs "rested" was no longer considered good treatment. Earl was very aware of this change from his reading in medical journals and contacts with other TB programs.

Robert Marks describes Earl in the 1970s as "the right person for the time," someone who was aggressive: "He had a good sense of the need for change." Earl was not always diplomatic, something that didn't change, but he saw "what had to be done," and he was "putting up with a lot of old customs." One of those old customs was rest therapy, and soon after becoming director, Earl ended this antiquated practice. The tradition in the TB ward at the Respiratory Hospital in Winnipeg had been that for large, scheduled parts of every day, the shutters and doors were closed, and patients had to rest. The nurses' job was to patrol the ward occasionally and make sure no one was breaking the rules and reading or doing anything. Here's what happened under Earl:

> I went into the wards as the new boss, and opened the doors – no more sleeping, no more resting, and the nurses didn't like that very much. We instituted a rehab program for the patients who'd been lying around for months wasting away, we started them playing basketball and volleyball, doing exercises. There were no more enforced rest periods with the doors closed.

But while some nurses were unhappy with the change, modern treatment of TB was going to mean increased responsibility and more challenging work for nurses.

Empowering nurses

Before the 1970s nurses were simply factotums, legs and hands to carry out the orders of omnipotent doctors, usually not even addressed by name ("nurse" was the universal tag). With the new technology of drug therapy for TB came a new division of labour that would directly affect nurses. Earl knew that drug therapy and the supervision of it were increasingly standardized, so that meant he could deal with more patients, and do his job more effectively, if he let nurses do more.

Nurses who worked with Earl from every phase of his career talk about how he respected their judgment and allowed them latitude to make independent decisions. But if he disagreed with your decision, you needed to launch a vigorous defense. It was no different in 1971, when Earl began working with Joann MacMorran, appointed in that year as the senior nurse in the TB control program. He laughs now about how he and MacMorran "fought every day," but he also says that he could not have run the program "without her fundamental agreement with my approach; she was the glue that put everything together." Earl believed from the beginning that TB control should be a "nurse-run" program:

> Nurses are the ones who have contact with patients. They need overall medical direction. Doctors should be on the periphery helping out. When you get doctors involved too much they tend to screw things up. They want to have control of meds, but they don't know how to deal with them. They don't know how to deal with adverse reactions. I started in Manitoba and many provinces have followed our model – central, run by nurses, with nurse-practitioners.

None of this meant that Earl wanted to see himself as Medical Director giving up control of clinical decisions: "I felt very strongly that the only way this was going to work was if we had central control by nurses with a physician director, with physicians working on the side." The nurses would communicate with each other more than with doctors, and "they would do contact follow-up, preventive treatment, and all the things necessary."

Earl describes himself as being very fortunate to have had only three nurses in the senior job as Nurse Consultant or coordinator: Janet Smith, who was in the job from 1956 until 1971; Joann MacMorran, from 1971 to 2002; and Nancy Williamson most recently. A lot of turn-over, Earl thinks, might have made him more hesitant to empower nurses as much as he did.

DRUG TREATMENT

The most important change for TB control in Manitoba from Earl's perspective was the new emphasis on drug treatment. "We thought that drugs were a good thing, not just a helper," says Earl. The 1953 film *The Road to Recovery*, made as an educational film in Manitoba for the Sanatorium Board, is a good indicator of prevailing attitudes when Earl took over. Drugs for TB are described in the narration as having "shown very encouraging results" and "tending to act as inhibitors to the growth of tubercle bacilli," when the reality was that these drugs were doing exactly what sanatoria never could: cure the majority of TB patients. But the film attributes merely "a powerful role in recovery" to drugs. To get beyond the sanatorium dogma you only have to read nurse Ethel Thorpe's version of events in Manitoba. Thorpe was a remarkable British woman who worked as a nurse consultant for four facilities operated by the San Board in the 1950s, including Ninette. In her master's thesis, which she completed at age 74, she recalls her early experience with drug therapy like this:

> I remember sitting in the Conference Room at Manitoba Sanatorium, Ninette, while Dr. A.L. Paine, the Med Super, showed me comparative x-rays of a patient before and after treatment with [the antibiotic] streptomycin. It was difficult to believe what we were seeing.

What they were seeing was, for the first time, a real cure for tuberculosis. Streptomycin would not be enough on its own, but by 1953 three of the major anti-TB drugs were available in Manitoba.

Earl says that in the 1960s "Manitoba was not very aggressive in the use of anti-TB medications. When I started in '64 there were even some patients who didn't go on drug regimens." Earl had been paying attention for some time to the studies done by the British Medical Research Council in India. He was aware of the multiple-drug regimens that were evolving to prevent drug resistance and cure TB. By 1967 all the drugs now in use except rifampin and its derivatives were on the market. The time had definitely come for Manitoba to start using drug regimens for all TB patients. Earl views this as the major achievement of his early years: "I instituted drug therapy as the main stay of the treatment of TB. If I had any contribution that was it – I insisted that people here in Manitoba got TB meds."

One reason that drug therapy was so difficult in the early years was that patients had to take huge numbers of pills for 18-24 months and then also get injections of the antibiotic streptomycin. A patient had to take about 19,000 pills for a complete treatment! Understandably, people did not always comply. Earl puts it this way:

> Nobody wants to take 19,000 pills. When they closed sanatoria all over the world, in the ceilings and behind the radiators, they found thousands of PAS pills [Para-aminosalisylic acid, a TB drug]. The drugs made you sick, and so people put them in their mouths and spat them out when the nurse left the room. That happened here in Manitoba too.

In the early 1970s, as more drugs became available, Earl started using "intermittent treatment." This was a regimen where patients took only two doses a week, but under supervision, so a nurse actually watched them swallow the pills. There were still unpleasant side-effects, but now there was no doubt that the medication was hitting its target. Also, this was a much easier regimen for the patients. They didn't call it "directly observed therapy," or DOT as it would later be called, but that's really what it was. Only some patients got it, the ones who they thought might not follow a regimen on their own. It would be more than 20 years before the World Health Organization recommended what was by then called DOT as the standard approach to treating TB.

The other drug-related innovation Earl introduced at this time was preventive therapy. Research had shown that the drug isoniazid (INH) could be used to prevent TB in patients who had had exposure to TB. The idea was that anyone who'd had contact with TB and was possibly harboring a latent infection would be prevented from getting active disease with this drug regimen. In the late 1960s when Earl started this in Manitoba, it was "a revolutionary idea." Now the United States Public Health Service and the Centers for Disease Control (CDC) in Atlanta consider such preventive therapy as the best way to eradicate TB, although the specific drug regimens have changed. Preventive therapy has been the focus of some of Earl's research work in Winnipeg for the CDC.

DEVELOPING A NEW PROGRAM

Just as drug therapy in Manitoba needed to fall into line with the leading practices in other jurisdictions, the same was true of other aspects of the TB control program. Without extended institutional care in the sanatorium, there would have to be new ways to identify people with TB, find and treat their contacts, and collect statistics on the disease.

Even apparently simple things like the Mantoux skin test for TB needed to be standardized in Manitoba. Earl says that as late as 1969, the province did not use commercially prepared tuberculin, but rather made its own. This had been the case for 30 years.

> It became obvious to me as the new boy on the block that nothing was standardized. So I said we have to investigate a tuberculin material that is the best one to use, and we tendered, and became like the rest of the world. There used to be various strengths, and so if you got a test result you didn't know if it was a 1, 5, 10, 100, 250 strength. So if you got a result in from somewhere you didn't know what batch they were using. Those kinds of data were hard to interpret.

CASE-FINDING

With the demise of sanatoria in Manitoba, it was essential to build some kind of infrastructure to control TB. Part of that infrastructure would have to be a method for "case-finding," or identifying patients with TB. In the old days the Sanatorium Board sent out trucks with x-ray equipment to do mass surveys in communities all over the province to find new cases of TB. Anyone with a positive diagnosis was sent to a san, very likely the one at Ninette. People also went to their physician, just like they do now, if they had a persistent cough, weight loss or fever; the doctor might diagnose them with TB, and then they'd be sent to the Central Tuberculosis Clinic in Winnipeg for an x-ray. From there, again, they mostly went out to the Ninette Sanatorium. Medical data on TB patients were kept in the Central TB Registry going back to 1926. But modern drug therapy had emptied the sanatorium beds and closed the institutions. The mass surveys were finding fewer and fewer cases of TB across the province. How would new cases of TB be identified now?

In the new era TB patients were still identified by case-finding teams from the Sanatorium Board, or diagnosed by a doctor and sent to the hospital. Case-finding though was now completely different. The modern jargon for the new method was "passive case finding" – but the process was far from passive. Instead of doing mass "surveys" of almost every community in the province, the Board's personnel now concentrated on the close contacts of people known to have TB. They were still called the survey team, but their work was now directed to very specific groups of people. Contact tracing was an important part of the new method, and it has changed very little since the 1970s.

Contact investigation was and is still done almost entirely by nursing staff and it is extremely labour-intensive. Nurses with many years of experience say it takes at least an hour for each patient. They need to become expert interviewers, develop trust and rapport with the patient, and have very good internal lie detectors. John Sbarbaro, an American doctor and pioneer in directly observed therapy (DOT) going back to 1966, jokes that "you have two minutes after you tell someone they have TB before they start lying." People lie about their contacts for obvious reasons – revealing them may be embarrassing, either because of the stigma of the disease, or because they have contacts they want to keep secret – lovers, visitors whose visas have expired, co-workers who will not be happy they came in contact with TB.

Contact investigation starts with the "presenting case," the person who has or is suspected of having TB. The idea is to find their contacts, screen them appropriately for TB infection and active disease, and then treat them as needed with drugs. The approach is also called concentric circle surveillance and it's often done by writing names and information in a circular pattern, sometimes on a pre-printed form. It's the epidemiological version of Dante's *Inferno*, with the inner circle being the hottest and most potentially hellish.

Concentric circle surveillance follows what doctors call the "stone-in-the-pond" principle, which means that the program screens the contacts of the presenting case in order of risk. Close contacts are in the first circle nearest the presenting case (the stone in the middle of the pond) and they need to be tested for TB infection first. These are high risk contacts, likely seeing the presenting case every day. Medium risk contacts see the patient about three times a week, and low risk contacts less than that. In order to classify the risk levels of contacts the nurse needs to find out how frequent and how long each of the contacts was, the size of the space where it occurred, and the quality of the ventilation. At a minimum, high risk contacts are given chest x-rays and skin tests for TB. The Nurse Consultant (or coordinator as the position was called) coordinates the tracing and testing process with input from the medical director.

One of the goals of contact investigation is to find the "index case" or source case, the TB equivalent of Typhoid Mary – the person who infected the presenting case. "Secondary cases" also need to be identified; they are patients who got infected from an identified source or index case. If a patient has been in a specific group while infectious, then everyone in that group needs to be tested if they were in close contact with the patient. Examples include a classroom, a bingo hall, an isolated First Nations community, or a group of people who drink together or sleep near each other in a homeless shelter.

"Absolutely centralized"

"SOME PEOPLE WOULD SAY IT WAS BECAUSE OF MY PERSONALITY, BUT WE RAN AN ABSOLUTELY CENTRALIZED PROGRAM. WE KEPT THE DOCTORS INFORMED. WE RAN A RIGID PROGRAM, AND THEREFORE WE GOT CONTROL OF TB." — EARL HERSHFIELD

The other big change was that with universal drug therapy for tuberculosis, and with full medicare funding for the medication in place by the early 1970s, it was essential for the TB control program to know who was taking exactly what drugs and when, and to get that information into the Central TB Registry. Patients with incomplete drug regimens might appear to get better but still harbour the TB bug, or even develop resistance to particular TB drugs, making them impossible or at least very expensive to cure. If patients had a prescription from their doctor and went to the pharmacy, they would have to pay for their TB meds. Doctors and pharmacists quickly learned that they could refer patients to Earl's program and get drugs to treat TB at no cost, but they had to cooperate with the program. If the doctor contacted Earl, he would exchange free drugs for information. Earl explains:

> I'd phone new doctors who didn't quite know the system and ordered drugs themselves, and say we need to keep records and follow up contacts … [so] it would be much easier if you could send us a little information, and we send the drugs out free. We rarely had any trouble after that.

With all this new information that needed to be recorded and centrally stored, it was inevitable as well that the Central TB Registry started to be computerized in the 1970s. Sophisticated relational databases would wait until the 1980s and 90s, but a punch-card system was in place very soon.

Five years into Earl's tenure as director, the provincial TB control system had evolved into what the Manitoba Department of Health and Public Welfare perhaps hoped for in 1928, when they received a committee report that recommended the "concentration of all tuberculosis activities in the province under a central authority." Although that had been true from an administrative point of view with the Sanatorium Board, it really only came true from a clinical viewpoint starting in the 1970s under Earl's leadership and initiative.

MAINSTREAMING TB

For Earl the major issue driving the closing of sanatoria was getting tuberculosis back into the mainstream of medicine. Earl recalls that in 1967 when he took over the program there were many professional meetings on this subject, and their common policy recommendation was to close the specialized TB institutions. One of the big issues was that people in sanatoria often had other diseases: diabetes, hypertension, cancer, and so on. With medical advances many of these diseases were now treatable, but not in sanatoria that were staffed by TB specialists and located far from mainstream hospitals.

"There was no reason," Earl says, "for a patient with TB and some other treatable disease to be sitting out there 120 miles from Winnipeg." In addition to needing access to a broad range of medical care, TB programs desperately needed modern facilities. Sanatoria, mostly built in the early 20th century, lacked isolation wards with negative pressure to prevent infectious TB patients from spreading the disease. Negative pressure ventilation equipment was new in the 1970s and it only existed in urban hospitals.

Earl readily admits that there was tension between the old guard and the young turks like himself: "I was the director of the TB program, so Dr. Paine, the director at Ninette, was literally under me, a guy who graduated with my father. I think it rubbed him a bit the wrong way that his classmate's son was now telling him what to do." But the closing of sanatoria was a national trend sweeping across the country, recommended by health policy consultants, and one that wasn't even that new by the early 1970s. Dr. George Wherrett had recommended the closing of sanatoria in his 1964 report for the Royal Commission on Health Services, with the only open question in his mind being that of timing. He took the major factors in closing sanatoria to be cost-driven and did not even mention the equally significant issue of generational change within the medical profession itself.

In 1967 a conference was held in Ottawa on "mainstreaming" TB back into the medical system, and the major policy recommendation from that conference was to close sanatoria. Earl was there, and he sees the event as a turning point for Canadian TB control. In the meantime there had been consultants in Manitoba looking at the sanatorium system and much correspondence between Earl Hershfield and Paine on the subject of closing Ninette. Soon mainstreaming TB "became the push of what was then called the Provincial and Territorial Directors of TB Control committee," which Earl sat on with his counterparts from other provinces:

> That's how the sanatorium movement ended. With the sporadic closing
> of sanatoria across Canada, each province at their own speed depending
> when people were retiring and beds in general hospitals were available.

Canadian health policy was changing dramatically in this period too, with medicare adopted in Manitoba in 1971, a year before the Ninette sanatorium closed. For many years if you had a positive x-ray for TB in a hospital, you literally were sent down a different hallway where all billings for your treatment were handled by a different system than if the x-ray had been positive for pneumonia, for example.

So really TB was being mainstreamed financially with the rest of the healthcare system. Canada followed Britain but with a huge time lag: by 1911 Britain had the National Insurance Act that provided free medical treatment, a maternity benefit and a 'sanatorium benefit' to insured workers. In Manitoba, there had been a separate private-sector fundraising system since the 1920s with the advent of Christmas Seals for tuberculosis treatment. Christmas Seals would continue, but from 1971 on all clinical services for TB patients – except Aboriginal people – would be covered by the provincially-run medicare system; Aboriginal

TB patients' services, like all their health care, would continue to be paid for by the federal government.

Mainstreaming TB meant closing institutions and building new ones that were more patient-centred. In a curious and unintended way it also meant making TB less visible. By 1975 the Sanatorium Board would be known to the public as the Manitoba Lung Association, and it would no longer run sanatoria or hospitals or operate large trucks to conduct mass TB surveys with. TB patients would go back to their homes and communities within a few months, cured. The absorption of the disease into the mainstream of medicine made TB easy to ignore, as did the success of Earl's TB control program. The resurgence of the disease in the 1990s, in Manitoba and all over the world, would serve as a stark reminder of why places like the Ninette sanatorium were built in the first place. Earl himself didn't need that reminder, as his commitment to immigrants with TB would show.

2

ROOTS

I t was no accident that Earl Hershfield became a doctor whose specialty was a disease afflicting poor people and immigrants. The Hershfield family fled anti-Semitic persecution in Ukraine and arrived in Winnipeg in 1910. Earl was born in 1934 on Selkirk Avenue, the heart of Winnipeg's legendary North End. Like so many other immigrants, the Hershfields were utterly determined to earn a place in Canadian society and to enjoy the freedom to practise their faith. Earl's father, Sheppy Hershfield, became a doctor in 1931 and was a well-respected family practitioner until his retirement in 1981. Longtime colleagues of Earl's, like Dr. Donald Enarson, an Albertan who is now the scientific director of the International Union Against Tuberculosis and Lung Disease, cite his father as Earl's overwhelming influence. Dr. Arnold Naimark, former president of the University of Manitoba and a friend of Earl's since childhood, says "I think a lot of his feel for the profession was instilled by his association with his father." Earl's father was far from being the only doctor in the family – Sheppy's brother Harry was too, and both of Sheppy's sons, Earl and his brother Melvyn became doctors.

Sheppy Hershfield published two memoirs. *I Remember When*, the first one, gives a vivid picture of the community that Earl grew up in: North End Winnipeg in the first half of the 20th century, and the Jewish community that was such an important part of Winnipeg history. Sheppy describes a North End farmers' market as a "colourful, noisy, smelly, exciting place," and pokes fun at the community's pretensions, noting that the Grand Opera House at Jarvis and Main was "neither grand nor [was there] any reason to call it opera." His stories of growing up in the North End display the same chutzpah and competitive zeal that his son Earl would later demonstrate in his professional life.

Even with Sheppy's zest for life, the anti-Semitism in the community could not be ignored, even if there were no pogroms. He describes harassment of Jewish school children and makes no effort to sugar-coat his experience. But for all the adversity, Sheppy was proud of his hardscrabble efforts to find a place in this new world:

> My years at Strathcona School are a treasure trove of wonderful memories of growing up in a difficult and often very antagonistic environment, of the many obstacles in the making of friends, of boys who would be bent daily on beating us up, of gradually finding one's way in the daily activities, in learning about sports and playing them and suddenly at the end of our stay at school to find ourselves the leaders, the sports heroes, the best students and having the grudging respect of students and teachers alike.

The most extended passages in the book are devoted to Sheppy's experiences as an athlete and as a newsboy on Main Street in front of the McLaren Hotel. Sheppy played baseball, soccer, and every other sport he could, but the greatest of these for him was baseball. He was an outstanding softball pitcher and instrumental in the founding of the local Young Men's Hebrew Assocation (YMHA).

Earl notes that "my uncle Leible, my father's youngest brother, was a tremendous athlete. He won many awards. He was invited to the Dodgers' training camp back in the '30s. His mother wouldn't let him go – he was 16 or 17." What is hard to appreciate in this day of the professional athlete and ubiquitous electronic entertainment is just how popular amateur sport was in Winnipeg in the 1920s and '30s. Hundreds of people attended baseball games that Earl's father pitched in, and people cared passionately about the outcome of these games. Many times games were sublimated versions of the tension between ethnic groups who populated the city: there were Irish teams, Scottish teams, French, Jewish, and Ukrainian. There was some pretty big-time gambling on some of the games too, and Sheppy recounts a story of being offered money to throw a baseball game in 1923, which he considered but declined.

Sheppy's account of his days selling newspapers reveals much about Winnipeg history but also a lot about his son Earl, who would never be noted for backing down or playing the wall-flower. Sheppy was an eye-witness to the most violent events of the Winnipeg Strike in 1919. He himself was ready to use his fists when it came to protecting his turf as a newsboy:

> There were the Shnider brothers who were stealing my customers. One day I beat up the older brother. They stopped selling papers to my customers. The Shnider brothers today are very successful business men in Los Angeles.

The outcome of many of Sheppy's stories that involve conflict or fighting is that his antagonist is defeated but goes on to succeed in life. Sheppy seems both tough-minded and tolerant, eager to see everyone claim their piece of the Canadian mosaic.

COMMUNITY

"I was born on Selkirk Avenue, the heart of the Jewish North End," says Earl, and that experience shaped him as much as his family life did. Earl was very much rooted in a community and a social circle:

> The friends that I made when I was 12 years old are still my friends today. It's a particular Winnipeg thing. I went to school with people who didn't move away, had similar interests. Also it didn't matter whether you were wealthy or not. We were very good friends because we all grew up together and had the same childhood experience, and we had the same interests in Winnipeg and in life.

Earl's father encouraged him to join the YMHA and through the 1940s and early '50s his social life revolved around it, with sports and dances and other events. A reunion in 1982 drew a thousand people, and Earl describes it as "one of the most wonderful days I've ever had in my life. You picked up conversations like it was yesterday." Earl's colleague Lee Reichman, who lives in New Jersey, says

> One of the things that's remarkable about him is he has the same social group that he grew up with. I think he's closer with people he's grown up with than just about anyone I've ever met. You know — she's a senator and so and so's something else. All these big wheels from Winnipeg are all in a single network, and they all have tremendous loyalty to each other.

Earl describes his rootedness in a community this way: "The people who we invited to meet our new friends were our old friends." Later when it came to choose where he would practise, Winnipeg was more attractive to Earl than the siren-song of bigger dollars in the United States.

LIKE FATHER...

"I've tried every sport, some I'm very good at, and others I'm not very good at," says Earl about his athletic career. Arnold Naimark remembers Earl as "a very good athlete" who competed in track and field, football, and basketball. Naimark managed the medical school's football team in the '50s, before there was intercollegiate competition at Canadian universities, and he says that Earl was "very fast... a great offensive back. I think he was good because he had a competitive streak, he pushed hard. I think the desire to succeed, to solve problems, was evident in his whole career."

Earl set a high school record for the 100 yard dash in 1951, so he was definitely fast, "but too small" for football. He remembers large crowds at the college football games and also at the YMHA baseball games where he played before college. Earl ended up playing baseball until 1988 when injury finally convinced him to hang it up. Like his father, he credits the game with introducing him to all sorts of people he would never otherwise have met. And competing was enjoyable.

For Earl, sports are also a model for handling conflict. When the game is over, no matter how hard fought it was, you shake hands and go home. When the meeting is over, no matter how much Earl yelled or criticized, you shake hands and go home. Conflict is an essential part of the game, but it's never about tearing people down. Earl puts it this way:

> I'm quick to anger and quick to forget about it. You cannot hold grudges otherwise you get into these horrendous fights, and nobody pays attention to the game anymore.

SOCIAL JUSTICE AND RELIGION

Earl Hershfield was raised in an orthodox Jewish home, and his father was "very imbued with Judaism." Dr. Anne Fanning, a TB expert who has known Earl for many years, talks about "his tremendous commitment to Judaism" and his interest in Jewish history. Earl describes himself this way:

> I am a believing Jew. Judaism is a liberal religion in the sense that we believe in social justice, and that's an integral part of our religion. My father of course was a strong believer in social justice for everybody.

For Earl medicine has never been about billing the most or publishing the most. Instead his belief in social justice led him to tuberculosis, a disease that Anne Fanning calls "so manageable and so poorly managed," a disease that mostly affects people in desperate need of social justice. Earl sees universal health care as a human right and something that is part of the Jewish belief system: "For hundreds of years in Europe we had organizations which looked after the health and welfare of the community. Every village and town had such an organization." In Winnipeg members of the Jewish community helped found institutions like Mount Carmel Clinic, which still serves the underprivileged, and built orphanages and senior citizens homes for their community.

Earl also sees his father's influence reflected in his own passion for social justice. The introduction to his textbook on TB control is dedicated "to the memory of my father, whose concepts of social justice for all had a profound influence on my life."

MEDICAL SCHOOL

Earl Hershfield went to medical school, as his father and uncle had, at the University of Manitoba. He met a nursing student named Betty Anne Fages, from Regina, Saskatchewan, and they got married in 1957. He graduated in 1958 with his MD and then worked as an intern and a resident at the Winnipeg General Hospital, the same hospital where he was born in 1934. Arnold Naimark describes him at the time as a "good, solid medical student," "very energetic," and "a quick study."

Earl was ambitious and wanted to be more than a general practitioner, so he would need more training. In 1960, Earl, Betty Anne, and their first son Jeffrey, moved to New York where Earl was to study pathology at Albert Einstein College of Medicine. As often happens, Earl changed his mind about his specialty, and decided that he was more interested in pulmonary (chest) pathology and lung disease. Then he moved to a chest hospital where many of the patients had tuberculosis, and this was his introduction to his life's work – although he didn't know it then. After a year there, Earl decided he wanted to do clinical medicine, and so he applied to the Mayo Clinic in Rochester, Minnesota.

While Earl studied in New York, the Hershfield family lived in the Bronx in an apartment only two blocks from the hospital where Earl was a resident. They had hoped for a holiday from Winnipeg winters but didn't get it – 1960 was one of the coldest winters on record in New York. Earl remembers that he got paid $2,000 for the year, from which he had to pay rent, car expenses and everything else for his young family. Finances were tight enough that they cashed in their empty Coke bottles a couple of times for the deposit money. "Once I found $20 in my pocket and that was gold in those days. I took everybody out to eat, the whole family for dinner." Earl's ability to enjoy life and still get his work done was already apparent:

> I'm a great baseball fan, and in pathology there are rarely any emergencies, so often on summer afternoons I'd check out and tell the hospital operator I'd call in every 25 minutes or so. Then I'd take the bus to Yankee Stadium. I used to watch the Yankees play – buy a cheap seat in the bleachers, but with the place almost empty I'd move down and get a great seat. I'd phone in to the hospital, say is anybody looking for me, are there any problems. Usually nobody was looking for me. I'd have a hot dog and Coke for lunch, and it was wonderful.

Earl's passion for sports helped broaden his social horizons. He remembers his friendship with Tom Casey, an African American medical student and former pro football player. He played for the Winnipeg Blue Bombers in the 1950s and ended up in the Canadian Football League's hall of fame. After his football career Tom became a doctor, studying with Earl in New York. Tom took Earl and Betty

Anne to a nightclub in Harlem called Small's, well-known because it was owned by basketball legend Wilt Chamberlain:

> Believe me we were the only two white people anywhere in Harlem. Tom introduced me to Wilt, who was seven feet tall and I was about five foot six. After hours the place became a jive club for the locals. We stayed there, we danced, drank and ate, and had a great time. Couldn't happen now, I don't think.

In 1961, Earl became a Fellow in Medicine at the Mayo Clinic Graduate School in Rochester, Minnesota, and so the Hershfield family moved there and rented a house. By now there were two sons, Jeffrey and David. Living in Rochester was a very different experience than life in the big city – Rochester was a small, well-to-do town where social life revolved around barbeques and movies. Other than the clinic the only major employer in Rochester at the time was IBM. The United States was emerging from the Korean War and the economy was booming; suburban communities like Rochester were growing rapidly. It felt safe and not a great deal different from living in urban Canada at that time. Earl notes wryly that "I say there were no problems but of course I was white, in a profession. Certainly there was the undercurrent of racism."

The stars in Minnesota were aligned in the right way to steer Earl towards a career in tuberculosis. The toughest and most interesting TB cases were referred to the Mayo Clinic from all over the state. Also it had been less than a decade since "Patricia T" came to the clinic and became world-famous as the first TB patient to be successfully treated with the antibiotic streptomycin. So, unsurprisingly enough, Earl's research project at the Mayo Clinic was about tuberculosis control. At the time he still thought of himself as a chest physician, an area that he "liked and had an aptitude for." So the stars were aligned but not yet easy to read.

ADVOCACY FIRST, DIPLOMACY LATER

"SUFFICE IT TO SAY I BELIEVED MY OWN RHETORIC, THAT TUBERCULOSIS CONTROL WAS IMPORTANT, THAT WE NEEDED TO DO IT, AND WE NEEDED TO DO IT RIGHT. MAYBE MY WAY WASN'T EVERYBODY ELSE'S, BUT I TRIED TO GET MY VIEW ACROSS SO EVERYONE KNEW WHERE I STOOD." — EARL HERSHFIELD

A mere four years after graduating from the Mayo Clinic, Earl was running Manitoba's TB control program. As the first chapter details, Earl's role was to be what MBAs call a "change-agent." Change is never painless, but Earl was both blunt and politically astute. He couldn't change things at the pace he might have preferred, but no one would ever accuse him of walking away from a fight he could win, either. His passion for social justice melded nicely with his absorbing interest in TB and its victims. Many doctors seem detached and even icy to the rest of us; that's not what Earl was like, then or now.

Meetings are a crucial part of the professional life of anyone who works in public health – this is the forum where major decisions are hammered out about policy and even individual cases. More than a dozen people who attended professional meetings about TB with Earl at the local, national, and international levels all said that Earl was emotional and even theatrical in meetings, but that it was because he cared so much about the issues at hand. In spite of the bluster, Earl would have a solid grasp of the facts, and he was a formidable opponent if you wanted to argue. At the same time, if you chose to disagree with him, he'd be perfectly friendly at the coffee machine afterwards, but still remind you that you were wrong.

Dr. Anne Fanning, a longtime colleague of Earl's who ran the Alberta TB control program from 1987 to 1996, says that "he was well regarded by everybody but with a sense that you wouldn't tread too lightly on that turf unless you were either nuts or you felt the issue was really relevant," and that his "rants were not devoid of reason." Earl himself puts it this way:

> I was passionate because I always wanted to make sure that decisions we made were reasonable, affordable, and not pie in the sky. I often become a devil's advocate simply to say there is another point of view. And I used to get passionate about it. I didn't always believe in what I was saying, but the decision-makers needed to understand that there might be a different point of view.

Fanning also remembers debates between Earl and Stefan Gryzbowski, who was the modern pioneer of TB research in Canada. Their debates about nuances of TB management looked so fierce to an outsider that you might have thought Earl and Gryzbowski hated each other. "The debate," says Fanning, "was always kind of a game." Fanning thinks that TB attracts people who get emotional about issues: "I get passionately involved in whatever I do, and I think that characterizes people who do TB."

Debates with Earl could be annoying to spectators or participants at times. Dr. Kevin Elwood, director of TB control for British Columbia since 1994, recalls one of Earl's tactics in meetings. "One of his great little tricks was he'd take out the *Globe and Mail* and start reading it if he didn't approve of any further discussion of a topic." But Elwood sees Earl as acting out of principle, not pique:

> He certainly had his views, and he wasn't afraid to be unpopular if he felt that what was being discussed wasn't appropriate. I guess people who weren't used to his style took it personally at times. But it wasn't about people – it was about the strength of his beliefs.

Dr. Brian Gushulak, now medical director for Citizenship and Immigration Canada, first met Earl in the early 1980s when he joined Immigration Health Services. Earl at the time was the respiratory disease consultant to the department. Gushulak says this about watching Earl perform in meetings:

> There are people who can be irritating, and people will end up not liking them. No one ever reacts that way to Earl even though he can be irritating and theatrical in meetings. His irritation is just a reflection of how he feels about the issue and it's not personal. People who've argued with Earl end up being his best friends.

> Whenever you have a difference of opinion with Earl it becomes an animated discussion. Earl gets red, and as he got older his hair was white, so you have this vision of a relatively short, not-skinny person becoming increasingly florid. That happened routinely.

Dr. Michael Iseman of the National Jewish Medical and Research Center in Denver, says that Earl "poked holes in people for getting a little too full of themselves," and that "although he was very serious he didn't take himself so seriously that he got full of himself." Iseman sees Earl as "a teacher to a whole generation of us working in the field of tuberculosis" both for his intellectual curiosity and his iconoclasm.

Brian Gushulak describes Earl as "the grand old man of tuberculosis in Canada." This is how he describes Earl's interest in immigrants and TB:

> There were others of his vintage who knew a lot about TB, but Earl had a profound interest in tuberculosis and immigration. He relates emotionally to the nature of the immigration process, since his own family were immigrants, and because of his professional interest in tuberculosis he was able to bring those two together. Earl was always a person who cared about the issue and in spite of his theatrical presentation he never carried a grudge.

People like Dr. Frank Plummer, now scientific director of the new Centre for Infectious Disease Prevention and Control in Winnipeg, identify Earl simply as "a Canadian icon" in the field of tuberculosis. Plummer jokes that medical residents at the University of Manitoba in the 1970s called him "Earl the Pearl," but the fact is that Earl is a rare breed. Very few Canadian doctors are left with his depth of experience with TB.

Before Earl there were other icons of TB control in Manitoba, most of them associated with the sanatorium at Ninette – David A. Stewart, Eddy Ross, Al Paine, and Tony Scott. They must have all sat in on their share of meetings and not always comported themselves with perfect dignity and detachment. What drove these doctors and their communities, leading them to build the TB control program Earl would inherit, is the subject of the next chapter.

3

END OF AN ERA

"SANATORIUMS HAD ABSOLUTELY NO EFFECT IN CURING TB. THE DEATH RATE
WAS ABOUT THE SAME. WHETHER TUBERCULOSIS PATIENTS WERE TREATED
IN A SANATORIUM OR NOT TREATED AT ALL, HALF OF THEM DIED."
— DR. LEE REICHMAN, *TIMEBOMB*

Tuberculosis left a distinct mark on the 19th and 20th centuries, and so did the sanatorium, the peculiar institution for treating TB that flourished all over the industrialized world. The story of the demise of that institution in Manitoba, its grassroots evolution, and its connection to developments in the rest of the world, is told here.

CLOSING NINETTE

Robert Marks, the Sanatorium Board's controller in the early 1970s, remembers that closing Ninette "was not without conflict," some of it driven by David Stewart, son of the David Stewart who was the Ninette San's founding director. By 1967 the Ninette sanatorium was the only remaining sanatorium in the province. Al Paine, the last medical director, had roots at the institution going right back to the 1930s when he worked under Stewart. So the Board waited for Paine's retirement in the summer of 1972 before they closed the sanatorium. Marks tells the story:

> I was the point man sent to close the sanatorium. They were down to about 90 staff. I called them all together and gave them notice. Jack Cunnings couldn't do it. He had been a patient there, and he said 'I'm too close to it.' It was a very emotional thing, just traumatic for these people, their world suddenly destroyed. It was a different world down there, totally removed from – well, almost from reality. You could live and die in that valley.

We had the employment services people out, but it didn't compensate for the trauma that the staff felt. At least one person had a nervous breakdown coming out of that, because what was he going to do — he wasn't that young. It was just the trauma of moving out of this institution that had looked after them for most of their lives. Many of the employees were ex-patients. They got the cure and they got a job, and then suddenly that's gone. It was very tense for a period of time. There was a lot of opposition to the closing, in the papers and so on. They weren't facing reality. The board took a lot of verbal brickbats.

In the end the Board did not sell the Ninette site, but instead operated the Pelican Lake Training Centre for mentally handicapped adults. This institution lasted until 2000, when these people too were mainstreamed into urban communities.

Ethel Thorpe explains very well in her 1989 master's thesis both what happened with the closing of Ninette and why it was to be so bitter for some of those attached to the institution:

As early as 1954, health service personnel were predicting there would be no need of sanatoria within ten years, and it became increasingly difficult to recruit doctors and nurses to staff such institutions.... A rear-guard of people remained.... A whole way of life for dedicated professionals, whose reward was in long-term personal relations with their patients, had gone with the advent of antibiotics. TB, which had been segregated on an emergency basis, had by the 1960s returned to the mainstream of medicine as the disease came under control, and it was difficult for many to believe that it had really happened. As with the buffalo, there was no return.

Now it is perhaps easier to see the closing of Ninette as part of a larger change in how TB was treated. Outpatient treatment of TB, with minimal hospitalization for the infectious, turned out to be more effective and cheaper than the sanatoria ever were, even once they had drug therapy available. Surgery, previously common for sanatorium patients, became a thing of the past.

Dr. Lee Reichman, director of the National Tuberculosis Center at the New Jersey Medical School, had an experience that's at least analogous to what happened in Ninette when he recommended closing the Glen Gardner sanatorium in 1974. It was the state TB sanatorium. There were protests and angry headlines in the New Jersey papers. Reichman says:

Sanatoria were often the biggest employers in a community. There were hundreds of them in the US. People have jobs, sometimes there's corruption involved. Everybody in the municipal government has someone on the san payroll, so the san is never going to go away. In New Jersey here they were afraid that the sanatorium director wouldn't be able to get another job, so they kept it open several years longer than they should have.

Communities became attached to sanatoria in ways that went much beyond their supposed medical purpose. With its long history, Ninette was the Taj Mahal of TB treatment in Manitoba, and nobody who drives a bulldozer up to such an institution will be universally loved.

Today you can take a tour of the few remaining buildings at Ninette conducted by someone from Youth for Christ, the new owners of the sanatorium site. Youth for Christ is renovating the buildings for use as a retreat and camping site. They've even created a little museum about the Ninette san in one room of the original 1909 building. There's an ancient defibrillator that looks like it was designed by a Chrysler engineer in the '50s, a huge silver sterilizing tank, and miscellaneous surgical equipment that looks distressingly primitive.

In one of the buildings you can see a row of chairs separated by a thick glass wall where sanatorium inmates could look at their loved ones without breathing on them. There are drawers for passing items back and forth but no speaking tubes. Maybe they used hand signals. Blood stains mark some of the walls, and some of the porches are unnaturally big to accommodate patients taking the open air cure for TB.

The legacy of the Manitoba Sanatorium at Ninette is partly in the bricks and mortar of this place. No one can help but be struck by how this beautiful site expresses the determination of the community to rid itself of a horrible disease. The modern campaign against TB in Manitoba will never have a tangible symbol like this.

BACK TO THE START

Early in the spring of 2004 I drive west on Manitoba provincial highway number 2 and then south on 18. Just before the two hour mark from Winnipeg you suddenly leave the flatland and descend into a lush valley and the town of Ninette. A mile east of town is the old sanatorium site. I keep driving south through Ninette and on into the small agricultural town of Killarney. I'm here to see Dr. David B. Stewart, long retired son of the original medical director of the Manitoba Sanatorium, whose name was David A. Stewart. David B. greets me outside his house, leaning on his cane and wondering if I have any objection to cats or pipe-smoking. I don't.

Dr. Stewart's book, *Holy Ground, The Story of the Manitoba Sanatorium at Ninette,* is the only concerted attempt anyone has made to write about the history of that institution, the embodiment of tuberculosis control for many Manitobans to this day. If you mention TB to any Manitoban over 50, and ask them to say the first word that pops into their minds, they will say "Ninette" or "the San." Many Manitobans who donate today to the Manitoba Lung Association's annual Christmas Seals campaign have no idea that the original name of the Lung Association was actually the Sanatorium Board of Manitoba. The Lung Association name change happened in 1975. Very few people realize as well that what is now called the Manitoba Lung Association bears responsibility for running the tuberculosis control program in Manitoba by an act of provincial legislation drafted in 1904.

Originally, the 1904 "Act Respecting a Sanatorium for Consumptives" did not provide as broad a mandate as what later evolved. But by 1928, the Act had been substantially amended, and soon the San Board, as people called it, was operating a central TB registry and a clinic in Winnipeg, mobile chest and x-ray clinics, a sanatorium with hundreds of beds in Ninette, and four other medical facilities that treated TB patients.

At the turn of the century tuberculosis was the leading cause of death in Canada, and something clearly needed to be done in Manitoba. In 1904, 24 prominent Winnipeggers were named to the Sanatorium Board. This act was unique in Canada; as David B. Stewart puts it to me in his dining room in Killarney:

> It made history because here was a volunteer board that had been entrusted with an entire public health program, empowered by act of legislature even though they were entirely a voluntary organization, the first of the NGOs in public health in Manitoba.

The San Board was indeed what we would now call an NGO, or non-governmental organization, but one that had an unusual government-provided mandate. Getting government funding would be a long and winding road, but where mandates exist, money tends to follow.

In 1909 the Board chose as a sanatorium site a 100 acre property that still sweeps picturesquely downhill to Pelican Lake just outside Ninette. The site apparently received the blessing of an official from the famous Trudeau sanatorium in upstate New York. By 1910 there were three large buildings and room for about 50 TB patients, with the men and women housed in separate "pavilions". The buildings were modeled after the Gravenhurst Sanatorium in the Muskoka region of Ontario. Eventually the sloping grounds would have 24 buildings, including a power plant, school, staff residences and 400 beds for TB patients – that's two buildings more than Trudeau's archetype in the Adirondack Mountains ever had, although Manitoba lacked the mountains. There was also a railway line that went out to Winnipeg dating back to 1898 when Ninette tried to become a big cottage community. Instead of cottagers, the CNR line brought patients, and over the years the lake got lower and greener with algae.

Earl Hershfield, who visited Ninette in the 1950s as a medical student, remembers that "the grounds were magnificent, with beautiful rolling hills and old wooden buildings kept in immaculate condition." He also remembers problems with the water supply and then the increasing number of empty beds through the 1960s. But, before the decline,

> The patients did very well. Many marriages, some children were born out of wedlock. Those people who lived and did well had a good life. The problem was many of them were there for years away from their families and their whole family life was broken up. Patients had to develop their own social life. The buildings were always clean and neat; I can remember every building was painted with a new coat of white paint every year. They had cottages for married people. Some of the people who were cured moved into the town of Ninette or up to Brandon, they didn't come back to Winnipeg.

In spring 2004, I walk through the empty former sanatorium buildings at Ninette on my way back to Winnipeg. David B. Stewart says that this place was the "valley of the shadow of death" for many of its inmates. I think about what it must have been like to be one of the many Aboriginal patients here in the 1960s, finally allowed into the big provincial San once it was falling apart.

BUILDING AN INSTITUTION

Dr. David A. Stewart was appointed by the Sanatorium Board as the first medical superintendent of the Ninette sanatorium in 1910, and he was in many ways perfectly qualified for the job. His family had wanted him to be a preacher, but he instead pursued medicine with a religious fervor. Stewart went into voluntary isolation so he could take care of patients stuck in the "pest house" during Winnipeg's great smallpox epidemic. He also worked part time through medical school as a reporter for the legendary editor John W. Dafoe at the *Winnipeg Free Press*. The last piece fell into place when he got TB himself and then took the cure at Edward Trudeau's famous Saranac Lake sanatorium in the United States early in 1910.

Initially Ninette's policy was to "to salvage the salvageable," in other words admit only those whose TB was not too severe. The idea was to save costs by avoiding patients who might need a protracted and expensive stay and likely couldn't be saved anyway. The British TB historian F.B. Smith notes that nearly all sanatorium directors had a published policy of admitting only "early cases." The belief was that a healthy san regimen could counteract the TB bug in these early cases and, besides, the cost of dealing with still-ambulatory patients was much smaller.

Unlike his British counterparts, Stewart took in the flood of advanced cases that arrived on the CPR trains. Many of the "salvageable" cases turned out to have long and distinguished careers working for the San Board. Bill Doern had wanted to be an electrical engineer before his admission to the San changed the course of his life in 1924. He played trombone at dances and parties at the San until a "double-pneumo" treatment left him with so little lung capacity he had to play a different instrument: he taught himself to play cello. With the advent of x-ray equipment at Ninette, Doern trained as a radiographer at the San. He went on to help start the Western Canada Society of Radiographers, and lived his whole life in the Ninette area, marrying another patient.

Evelyn McGarrol, now 101 years old and living in a seniors' residence in west Winnipeg, remembers with perfect clarity being diagnosed with TB and sent out to Ninette in 1928, where she stayed for 16 months. By 1930 she was a secretary at the Central Tuberculosis Clinic, a position she held through the first year of Earl Hershfield's tenure in 1967.

Jack Cunnings is perhaps the most prominent example of a former patient who went on to work for the Sanatorium Board, eventually becoming executive director. When Cunnings became Rehabilitation Director at the Central Tuberculosis Clinic in 1942, his thinking was right in line with Stewart when it came to rehabilitation of long-term patients. Stewart talked about "redeeming the time," by which he meant finding something useful to do that would prepare the patient for life back in the outside world. The San had a school for children starting in 1925 and also did vocational training from early on. There was a rehabilitation officer who helped patients plan careers "in keeping with their capacities," which usually meant needlework, woodwork, or watch repair. Many of these programs were clearly modeled on ones run in Britain for TB patients starting in the 1930s. Stewart and Cunnings recognized that people who were out of the workforce for months or even years would need support programs to get their lives re-started, and also that people with jobs were less likely to get sick again.

SANTHROPOLOGY

David B. Stewart's book *Holy Ground* is as much a memoir of sanatorium culture in the first half of the 20th century as anything else, although it is written mostly from an institutional perspective. Stewart, who grew up in the Ninette institution that his father ran, writes a little about his own experience. For example, he waxes poetic about the San's power house, "a boy's paradise…. Even yet in my dreams I sometimes revisit the sprawling building which included the laundry, engine room, boiler room and repair shops." He describes the Sanatorium Orchestra that he himself played in, and the New Year, Summer Picnic, Thanksgiving, Halloween, and Christmas celebrations that took place.

Even with special events and educational programs in full swing, long-term patients had an enormous amount of time to kill. Stewart describes the installation of a public address system in 1929 that broadcast radio programs and even the World Series. There were limits to how much culture a doctor could take:

> ... after lunch and in the early evening, records were sometimes played
> [over the P.A.]; but that was strictly regulated. Dr. Stewart disliked jazz,
> and if something played that he didn't like the operator usually had a
> grumpy telephone call from the house on the hill.

The Board's 1953 educational film on TB, *The Road to Recovery*, comes from the second-last decade of the Ninette San. It conveys with dogmatic energy the unchanging sanatorium message: the only way to a cure for the tuberculous is through the sanatorium. There are no other roads or gods. In the film, Aboriginal people are visible only in racially segregated environments, and not at Ninette. There are shots of the well-coiffed grounds and the buildings, and special events like the visit of Santa and Mrs. Claus at Christmas. The film clearly lays out the standard treatment program, which consists of rest, diet, drug therapy, and surgery.

"John," the fictional patient whose progress the film follows, is sent to Ninette with no worry about hospital bills; how much income John will lose is unmentioned. The overwhelming emphasis of the narration is on the importance of rest and routine. Patient docility is taken for granted, even though it could not be in real life:

> Every new patient in a sanatorium has a whole new routine to learn, a
> routine that's aimed at getting the maximum benefit from each day. Out
> of it comes a knowledge of how to live in bed and like it, so peace of
> mind is also quite essential.

Bed rest, the narration goes on, "remains the foundation of treatment on which all others depend for ultimate recovery." There's also a scene in which Dr. A.L. Paine, last medical superintendent in Ninette, enters a room of nurses. They all stand, as if he were a visiting head of state. I described this scene to a Manitoba doctor whose career began in the 1960s, and he commented, "it was a period when doctors were very paternalistic. Patients lost their freedom in the sanatorium. Their hopes and dreams and lives were often over."

THE COST OF GROWTH

Whatever doubts hindsight confers on the sanatorium regimen, Ninette's institutional story is one of almost continuous growth. "We are overwhelmed by our very success," David A. Stewart wrote in 1927, a year after the Christmas Seal campaign had helped the Board purchase portable x-ray equipment and start conducting mobile TB clinics. The advent of traveling clinics led to a problem common in the early history of any public health program: the number of TB cases skyrocketed. The trend continued in 1929 when the Board acquired a Ford van with a small Delco generator that allowed the clinics to travel, for the first time, to communities with no electricity.

More x-rays and exams produced more patients for the sanatorium, and more patients meant higher operating costs. Tuberculosis also became a notifiable disease by law in 1934 in Manitoba, putting further pressure on the Board to find all TB cases. Again the British influence was apparent, as Britain had compulsory notification by 1913 to prevent the spread of the disease.

Funding for the San, which was tenuous at the beginning, became increasingly difficult. The Tuberculosis Control Act of 1929 made the Board responsible for coordinating TB control throughout the province. With the country going into the Great Depression as well, Stewart wrote in 1933 about Ninette's financial struggles:

> ...the difficulties are such that the whole question of the basis of payment for the care of tuberculous people has to be reconsidered without delay in order that doors be kept reasonably open. Costs are beyond revenues and have been for some time.

In the 1930s the Union of Manitoba Municipalities brought in a levy paid to the San Board that amounted to a form of medical insurance: now all TB patients who couldn't pay for their treatment at sanatoria would be covered. But this levy was not enough. Ninette's spacious grounds now included vegetable gardens, potato fields and a piggery, all designed to lower food costs. Winnipeg started paying for the treatment of its citizens in the 1940s, and there was a guarantee of federal funding for war veterans by then.

Also in 1930 the Sanatorium Board opened the Central Tuberculosis Clinic, or CTC, at the corner of Bannatyne and Olivia Street in Winnipeg. Dr. Tony Scott was put in charge. Then there were other facilities whose work needed to be coordinated and tracked for the central tuberculosis registry maintained at the CTC. One of them was the old King Edward Hospital, dating back to 1912 and operated by the city of Winnipeg. Then in 1931, the St. Boniface Sanatorium opened at St. Vital, run by the Grey Nuns.

By 1939 the Board was also operating the Dynevor Indian Hospital just north of Selkirk under a contract with the Department of Indian Affairs. It was small but also the first sanatorium for Aboriginal people in Manitoba. The site was a converted Anglican church hospital. The Board took on another Indian Affairs contract in 1945 to run Clearwater Lake Sanatorium near the Pas. It was a former US Air Force base. Two years later the Board began running the Brandon Sanatorium, which was converted from a Canadian Air Force hospital to what was then called an Indian hospital. All of these institutions segregated Aboriginal people from white patients, who were treated in larger better-equipped facilities.

This expansion was costly, but the champions of sanatorium care argued that the per patient cost was much lower than the cost of putting patients in a general hospital, and this was perfectly true. The brutal and unexplored reality, however, was that tuberculosis patients were just as likely to die or recover if they stayed home. And of course the cost to the patients, in terms of lost income, lost relationships, disruptions of family life and career, was never calculated. The only guaranteed benefit of the sanatorium was that your family, friends, and co-workers were less likely to catch the disease from you, provided they didn't visit too often or get too close when they did.

Surgery was to become a central focus of the Manitoba Sanatorium. Again this was not an innovation, but an adoption of well-established European and American trends towards what were called "modern" sanatoria, which did not simply provide cottages and rest but also dramatic surgical interventions that might stop the dreaded disease.

RADICAL INTERVENTIONS

"YOU HAVE TO APPRECIATE THAT IN THE 1940S, YOU HAD ABOUT A 60% CHANCE OF BEING DEAD IN FIVE YEARS FROM TB, SO THE DISEASE GENERATED SOME RADICAL, IN RETROSPECT SOME CRAZY THINGS IN PURSUIT OF A CURE."
— DR. MICHAEL ISEMAN, PROFESSOR AND TUBERCULOSIS SURGEON AT
NATIONAL JEWISH HOSPITAL, DENVER

"The sanatorium has at length become a specialized hospital," wrote a British doctor in 1938. The main specialty was collapse therapy for the lungs, a whole set of surgical techniques that collapsed the lung in order to "rest" it, and Ninette's sanatorium provided the whole gamut of tuberculosis surgery for almost 50 years, starting in 1914 with the artificial pneumothorax procedure.

For many patients at Ninette, surgery meant artificial pneumothorax, whose purpose was to "compel it [the lung] to rest," as the narrator puts it in the 1953 film The Road to Recovery. The procedure was far from restful from a patient's viewpoint. The chest was pierced in front with a hollow needle after a local anaesthetic was administered. Then the surgeon would pump air into the pleural cavity, the space between the lung and the chest wall, in order to collapse the lung. This was repeated a few times. A few hours after the initial procedure, a patient reported feeling "knifelike pains in the chest" which "continued for three days and nights." After that, "refills" were needed to keep the lung collapsed, with a regular schedule of these procedures over a three or four year period. In many cases (documented in Britain, but not at Ninette), the needle perforated the lung. 50% of British pneumothorax procedures were followed by pleurisy, and occasionally there was "pleural shock" and death. A British Medical Research Council investigation in 1922 found that half the patients were dead within three years of receiving a pneumothorax procedure. No statistics of this kind were kept at Ninette.

David A. Stewart had been skeptical about the more radical surgeries in the early years at Ninette. However, when his wife got very sick with TB and couldn't be treated with pneumothorax, he took her to Montreal for surgery around 1924, where she had 50 inches of rib removed on one side (a thoracoplasty). She then lived another 12 years, and so Stewart decided that these kinds of surgeries might have a place as last-ditch efforts to save those who couldn't be helped any other way.

The Road to Recovery gives what may be the best official picture of surgery at Ninette. Surgery is presented as an essential component of the cure, and by 1953 drug treatment was considered "particularly valuable before and after surgery," but strictly an adjunct to the whole san regimen. John, the film's model patient, has a team of doctors who consult and come to what appears to be a foregone conclusion: John needs surgery.

Sometimes the doctors at Ninette decided a patient needed permanent collapse of the lung. For this there was plombage, described in *Holy Ground* like this: "the lung was compressed by stuffing the inside of the chest wall with some inert material, usually paraffin wax." Other jurisdictions used ping pong balls.

Ethel Thorpe, a nurse consultant for the San Board in the 1950s, wrote about the Ninette TB surgeries in her 1989 master's thesis:

> Some of these operations took eight hours to perform, required continuous blood transfusion for the patient throughout, and eight hours of continuous anaesthesia…. There was no such thing as intensive care units…. The post-operative care of these patients required dedicated skill from surgeons, physicians, and nurses under conditions that would today be considered unbelievable.

I found a ledger at the Sanatorium Board's Winnipeg offices called a "Register of Operations" from Ninette for the period January 1956 to 1970. There is a clear declining trend: in 1960 there were 79 "major" surgeries, including 7 wax packs or plombage procedures; in 1965 there were 57 major surgeries; in 1969 there were 7 surgeries in total, and by 1970 there were none. The information in this register is extremely minimal. For example, an entry for November 7, 1960, lists the patient's name, the procedure, and the "postoperative condition." The procedure is listed as "thoracoplasty, four ribs left," and the postoperative condition is described as "good." Every single one of the hundreds of major surgeries in this register is described with a "good" postoperative condition. If there were any bad ones, no one was counting.

Earl Hershfield says that "we stopped surgery at Ninette because they didn't have an intensive care unit, or the background to do major lung surgery. I was instrumental in reducing surgery out there." Patients who still needed surgery came into the Winnipeg General Hospital, with its modern operating room and fully equipped intensive care unit.

A SHORT HISTORY OF THE SANATORIUM BUSINESS

The tuberculosis treatment program at Ninette emphasized fresh air, rest, wholesome diet, and specialized lung surgery, and none of this program was unique to the Manitoba institution. Instead it was rooted in the international sanatorium movement and the history of TB treatment. This movement was astonishing in two ways: for its massive institutional success and its equally large medical failure. At no point before the modern drug treatment era did sanatoria manage to avoid the deaths of roughly half their patients, and that's without counting the relapses whose cases were not tracked. Yet institutions like Ninette provided palliative care, brought communities together to build lasting institutions, and often gave hope where there was little cause for it. Some of their surgical interventions had positive effects as well as providing new knowledge for treating various lung diseases. And no modern immunologist would argue against the benefits of peace, good diet, and fresh air.

One of the features of the original buildings at Ninette was the large open air balconies where, except in the dead of winter, patients slept and rested outside to get fresh air. Fresh air was considered an important part of curing TB in sanatoria. A doctor in Winnipeg recently told me this story about the rigours of taking the cure:

> She [his patient] was in the sanatorium at Ninette, and even as late as when the modern drugs were available, in the 1950s, patients were expected to sleep outside in winter weather. She described wrapping herself in what was called a Klondike blanket. If you had to get up to pee in the middle of the night, it was a real nightmare wrapping yourself up again.

Tuberculosis treatment before the antibiotic era was an inexact science, largely because there was no reliable cure. So even though doctors had understood it was an infectious disease since Koch's discovery in 1882, many earlier practices survived. The obsession with fresh air went back to the practice of climatology, a pseudo-science whose roots extend back even earlier than the first sanatoria. Climatology's premise was that a change in climate could cure or at least ameliorate certain ailments.

In the 19th century British doctors could well have had side-businesses as travel agents. They recommended foreign destinations for TB patients based on the stage of their disease. Sea voyages were healthy for early stages, and once you looked anorexic it was time for southern Italy. If you were rich, horseback riding and skiing were supposed to be good.

However, any doctor is likely to at least attempt managing a disease, and so in the absence of effective treatment it was inevitable that a form of institutional care for tuberculosis would arise. Doctors gradually lost their enthusiasm for particular climates and locations as possible cures as these new institutions were established. The first sanatorium for the treatment of tuberculosis in the open air was the Royal Sea Bathing Infirmary for Scrofule (scrofula, a form of TB), organized in 1791 in London by a fashionable Quaker doctor. Like most early sanatoria, this institution catered to those with money, and resembled a luxury spa. Andrew Nikiforuk, in his essay on the history of TB, writes that "before Club Med, there was Club TB." But the disease was killing so many people that there would be relentless pressure to expand the club.

The sanatorium era began in earnest with a German doctor named Hermann Brehmer, who founded an institution in 1859 that promoted a TB cure based on fresh mountain air, healthy diet, rest, and supervised exercise in the form of mountain walks. Brehmer believed that TB was caused by poor blood circulation to the lungs, and that it could be cured by exercise at high altitude and an enriched diet to stimulate circulation. The Silesian Alps, now part of Poland, were an ideal location for providing this treatment, and his whole program rapidly became famous. Germans were already accustomed to going to spas for health reasons, and so the Brehmer sanatorium was just an extension of an established cultural practice. Brehmer's assistant and ex-patient, Peter Dettweiler, ran a sanatorium in the mid-1870s that put much more emphasis on close medical supervision and resting in open balconies. It too was very influential, helping to change TB treatment methods in Britain in particular. British doctors at institutions like the Brompton Hospital (1841) had provided palliative care and very little therapeutic intervention. With the German influence, they began to order rest for TB patients who were sick and feverish, and exercise for patients who were feeling better.

The German influence also extended to Switzerland, which soon became the centre of the world's most glamorous sanatoria through the late 19th century. The most famous of the Swiss sanatoria were in Davos starting in the 1870s. Thomas Mann's novel, *The Magic Mountain,* is set in a Davos sanatorium, where the main character stumbles into a seven year "cure" for TB when he is supposed to be merely making a visit. Like most Swiss sanatoria until 1939, this one was more a hotel than a hospital. When the Swiss brought in more doctors to do residential treatment of TB, medically supervised rest cures became so entrenched that Swiss doctors resisted drug therapy well into the 1950s.

The Swiss economy was sharply boosted by the sanatorium industry. Sanatoria were so popular with the wealthy that the country's banking and pharmaceutical industries directly benefited. Sanatorium patients needed banking services to stash away their money as they lay dying. Then they needed drugs, and the infant drug industry was willing to make sales before effective products existed. When TB did come under control with drug treatment, sanatoria were, with wonderful practicality, turned into ski resorts. Davos is now famous for its summit meetings on world economics, and few visitors remember why some of the balconies are so large. On the other side of the ocean, many winter sports facilities in Colorado, Nevada, and Arizona have the same origins.

In Britain, birthplace of socialized medicine, the health authorities began building sanatoria for middle income and even poor people by the 19th century. Unsurprisingly, some doctors decided that poor people could best be cured by supervised ditch-digging and other labour. But on the whole rest therapy prevailed for all classes, although sanatoria for the poor were more highly regimented and frequently under-staffed and poorly heated (cold was supposed to be good for TB patients anyway). By the end of the 19th century there were 17 specialized hospitals to treat TB in Britain, with about 1,100 beds; though they were not called sanatoria, they were really an industrialized version of the now-familiar institution. In addition, by 1911 there were 108 sanatoria in the British Isles.

The sanatorium movement came to North America largely because of one doctor, Edward L. Trudeau. Dr. Peter Warren, a medical historian at the University of Manitoba, summarizes what happened:

> Trudeau went out to the Adirondacks in New York when he came down with tuberculosis. He went shooting and fishing, which he enjoyed, and didn't die of his TB. At some point he started to read literature in medicine and discovered these German-Swiss sanatoria. He thought, here I am in the mountains in the cold fresh air and I'm doing very well. So he opened a sanatorium that became a mecca for everyone in TB to go and study and the whole sanatorium movement in North America came from that.

Trudeau's sanatorium opened in 1885 and was called the Adirondack Cottage Sanatorium. It was located at Saranac Lake, and the one ongoing legacy of the institution is the Adirondack chair, originally invented to accommodate a TB patient stretching out almost horizontally in fresh air. With funding from wealthy acquaintances, Trudeau provided cottages for those who could not otherwise have afforded care. He also ran a laboratory and was an enthusiastic if unproductive scientist. None of the real breakthroughs in tuberculosis treatment would come from his or any other sanatorium.

However, when Dr. David A. Stewart of Manitoba became ill with TB in 1910, he headed to Trudeau's treatment mecca on Saranac Lake. Doctors were treated at no charge, but the value of what Stewart learned there was incalculable to him: the treatment regimen, and institutional life were a prototype for the new Ninette San on Pelican Lake. There may not have been mountains, but the air was fresh, often cold, and the lake was the largest navigable body of water in southwest Manitoba.

South of the border the United States had followed Britain in converting hospitals into TB institutions, and by 1950 there were over 100,000 beds available for TB patients. Many of these sanatoria charged patients only what they could afford to pay. Sanatoria were so ubiquitous they even had an impact on interior design: linoleum became popular because flooring salesmen claimed it prevented the transmission of TB germs hiding in floor cracks. There were thousands of sanatoria all over the world, many built with money contributed by Christmas Seals fundraising and cherished by the often remote communities where they were located.

Canada's first sanatorium was the Muskoka Hospital, which opened in 1897 in Ontario. Kentville followed in 1904 in Nova Scotia, Ninette in 1910, and the Fort Qu'Appelle Sanatorium ("Fort San") opened in Saskatchewan in 1917. Many former military hospitals were converted into sanatoria in all the provinces — in the Maritimes, Alberta, B.C. (Nanaimo and Prince Rupert), and in Manitoba with Clearwater Lake near the Pas, and a Canadian Air Force hospital at Brandon.

The classic history of tuberculosis in Canada, George Wherrett's *The Miracle of the Empty Beds,* came out in 1977 and still bears the heavy imprint of the sanatorium era. He credits Hermann Brehmer's German sanatorium with "establishing ... the value of open-air treatment," and tells what he saw as a story of continuous progress towards the antibiotic-enabled miracle of the 1950s.

The prairie provinces led the country in their zeal to establish bricks and mortar to defeat TB, as Wherrett notes:

> At one stage in the program it was thought that enough sanatoria could be developed in Canada to treat every case of tuberculosis. This actually happened in Saskatchewan, Manitoba, and Alberta, but in the other provinces it was not until the drug era that there was a sufficient number of treatment beds.

Beds and bricks, as it turned out, were not always going to be useful; the new TB drugs emptied beds and closed institutions through the 1960s and into the '70s. The bricks and mortar of the sanatoria were gone, and even the word tuberculosis gradually disappeared: lung disease and respiratory medicine were what people saw and talked about. Earl sums up the later 1970s like this:

> A decline in the disease rate of 7% per year was acceptable, and nobody was too excited about it. I was looking for other things to do, so I joined the Lung Association in Ottawa, and we began to branch out into tobacco, cancer and all the other things and that's what everybody did. Public health programs across the country disappeared or were made much smaller.

Nobody would have guessed in 1975 that tuberculosis would still fiercely live on into the new century and at alarming rates in some parts of the province. In fact, TB's creeping resurgence would be invisible to most of Manitoba's citizens in 2005.

4

TB 101

To understand TB's global resurgence, you need to understand a little about the disease and its history. This is, after all, a disease that is treatable and curable but still kills two million people per year. Without understanding the history of TB treatment, it's very difficult to understand TB's interrelationship with the AIDS crisis, the problem of drug resistance, and why TB is once again out of control.

Getting TB is not difficult. All you have to do is breathe in TB germs from someone who's infectious. No one knows exactly how many TB germs someone usually inhales to get the disease, but a few droplets containing the bacteria will sometimes infect you. It's also easy to develop resistance to the drugs used for TB treatment — all you have to do is fail to take all your pills; the average treatment now lasts six to nine months, and taking all those pills after you've started feeling better is very hard, especially when the pills are tough on your system. Many people can't afford the drugs or can't get access to a clinic. Dying of TB is easy too, especially if you have AIDS already sabotaging your immune system. Having both diseases is a death sentence for the millions of people who are not getting treatment.

Pulmonary tuberculosis is a lung disease and the most common form of TB, and the only kind that's infectious. It can eat holes in your lungs so they no longer supply oxygen and you eventually choke to death. Here's how it works. You breathe TB germs, or bacilli, in from someone who has the disease who coughs or sneezes around you. The germs come through the windpipe to the lungs. The lobes of the lungs are like sponges filled with air spaces, and these air spaces are called alveoli. The alveoli exchange oxygen from the incoming air for carbon dioxide, the waste product of human respiration. Your body's first defence cells against the germ invaders are called macrophages, and they try to swallow the TB germs as if they were playing Pacman. But that is not easy. The tuberculosis germ or bacillus has a waxy, tough coating that makes it difficult to absorb and also allows it to hang around in the dust or the air. Any bacteria are most vulnerable to the body's defences when they reproduce. But unlike more common bacteria, which reproduce every 20 minutes or so, the TB bacillus only reproduces every 24 hours.

In spite of the unusual toughness of TB bacteria, 90% of people who get primary infection do not become ill with the disease. Instead, the body's immune system controls the TB germs. Even if you do get TB, there are usually no symptoms at all in the early stages, making it hard to diagnose. By the time you are coughing, having fever, night sweats, or even spitting up blood from your lungs, you have an advanced stage of TB. Then, of the fortunate 90% of infected people whose immune systems control the TB bugs for a while, a small group of them will still get the disease – it can lie dormant for years and then suddenly make you ill.

But you may be among the unlucky 10% of the population that gets TB within two years of being infected. In this case your body's defences don't succeed in killing the invading bacilli early on, you aren't treated with germ-killing drugs, and then the TB germs actually break into the macrophage cells and multiply inside them. The germs create a tiny nodule that's like a tumor and called a tubercle, from which the disease gets its name. The TB germs metastasize a bit like cancer does. It takes millions of TB bacteria to make a hole, or cavity, in your lung. These holes damage your ability to breathe and circulate oxygen to your body. They show up on chest x-rays. The holes look like black spots on wispy white clouds over the lung. If the TB germs keep multiplying and the holes in the lungs keep growing, your respiratory system is impaired and will eventually stop working.

The time it takes before you have a serious respiratory problem varies a lot. In Victorian England they talked about "galloping consumption," which consumed patients rapidly, making them lose weight and finally choke to death, at a galloping pace. Other patients cantered in a more leisurely fashion to their deaths or recoveries. TB patients lose colour as well, which is why the disease was often called the "white plague," as in the title of René Dubos' famous 1952 book on tuberculosis. Nowadays people who get co-infected with HIV and TB are very likely to get galloping consumption; someone with full-blown AIDS and TB has an average lifespan of five weeks.

TB can also infect the bones instead of or in addition to the lungs. One of the most common infections is now called Pott's disease, and it deforms the upper spine into a curve. The ancient Egyptians considered tuberculous hunchbacks to be holy, and preserved their bodies as mummies. TB can also infect the kidneys and the gastrointestinal tract. One other non-infectious form of TB is scrofula, where the lymph nodes on the side of the neck swell up with infection. These sores were called "the king's evil" in England and France, and people stood in line by the hundred to be cured by the king's touch. This cure was so popular you had a good chance of being trampled in line before the king ever touched your sore. Scrofula is rare now, but it was once commonly caused in children by unpasteurized or impure milk.

TB SYMPTOMS

More than 90% of people who get infected with TB have no symptoms initially. But the fact that they have been infected is revealed when they test positive on a tuberculin or Mantoux test. The tuberculin test or skin test consists of injecting a substance containing material from the cell wall of the TB pathogen into a small patch of the patient's arm skin. If there is swelling of 10 millimetres or more in 48 to 72 hours, the test is considered positive, although swelling of 5 millimetres is enough to be considered positive if the patient has HIV or is a close contact of someone with infectious TB.

The next step for someone who tests positive is to get a chest x-ray or have a sputum sample examined under a microscope. Diagnosing TB is often a combination of science, art, and detective work. The detective work might include knowing that someone came to Canada from a country where TB is prevalent, or has had previous treatment for TB, or has Type II diabetes, or a damaged immune system, or is homeless or an intravenous drug user — any of these things should raise suspicion. The scientific part of diagnosis always includes lab work. Joyce Wolfe, who manages the national reference lab for TB at Winnipeg's Microbiology Laboratory, says that TB bugs are extraordinarily hard to work with:

> Its characteristics make it a difficult organism to isolate from a patient sample. There's countless other non-TB bugs in any sputum sample. Your goal is to get rid of all the other bacteria and keep the TB intact so you can grow it. The harsh methods you have to use to get rid of bacteria also are hard on the TB germs. In the lab it's quite a procedure – it takes about an hour and a half to process one sample. So for a patient who has just a few TB bacteria, it's difficult to isolate. You need a really good lab to do this in.

Regardless of whether lab work is done, once TB is more advanced people start to show symptoms. They may have a persistent cough, fevers, fatigue, and extreme weight loss. If someone coughs blood like the English romantic poet John Keats did, they have a very bad case of standard-issue pulmonary TB. It is possible to get a horrible and unpredictable diarrhea from gastrointestinal TB. Then there is tuberculous meningitis in children, which if untreated with TB drugs, is almost always fatal. But pulmonary TB – tuberculosis in the lungs – accounts for 75% of active disease cases.

Dr. Michael Iseman, a TB expert at the National Jewish Medical and Research Center in Denver described to me how doctors understood pulmonary TB, quite correctly, before 1950:

What the old-timers taught us about TB was that the cavity in the lung was the epicentre of the earthquake. In the cavity the bacteria grew exponentially, and within the cavity there may be a billion or ten billion bacilli, and it was where you had large populations that were rapidly multiplying. Here the lottery of drug resistance was active; with a large number of active organisms, mutations that would spawn the next generation of drug resistance were much more likely to occur. The whole balance shifts biologically between the infection and the host. TB is kind of like an avalanche once it begins. Cavities form, fevers occur, weight loss occurs, malnutrition intervenes, immunity gets worse and pretty soon you're tipped over and on a rapid path to death and consumption.

A SHORT HISTORY OF TB

Tuberculosis is the oldest known infectious disease that affects human beings, but recent evidence suggests it only began to affect us about 15,000 years ago. It's part of a 300-million-year-old germ family called mycobacteria, the same class of organism that causes leprosy. Both TB and leprosy are chronic diseases that destroy tissue: leprosy destroys skin and nerves, and TB damages lungs and sometimes other parts of the body such as the brain, kidneys and bones.

There are three main kinds of TB bacteria that affect humans. The type spread by humans themselves is called *Mycobacterium tuberculosis,* and it is the most common. The bovine variety *(Mycobacterium bovis)* is spread by infected cattle but has stopped being a problem where milk is pasteurized and the health of cattle carefully monitored. The avian type *(Mycobacterium avium)* is carried by infected birds but does occur, on occasion, in humans, especially in those who are HIV-infected.

The Greeks and Romans built early cities, lived close together, and coughed frequently with TB. They called the coughing sickness *phthisis,* pronounced "tea-sis". Hippocrates, the doctor with the famous oath, thought phthisis was an incurable disease and the most fatal one he'd encountered. With rare professional candour, he recommended leaving patients in the late stages of the disease alone, as attending would only hurt a doctor's reputation. The Roman physician Claudius Galen also considered TB incurable. Since the disease was common in the Roman empire, he quite sensibly suggested good food and fresh air. Later doctors would advocate everything from warm climates and the pseudoscience of "climatology" to more actively harmful practices like blood-letting and injecting gold salts.

Mycobacteria have the potential to destroy any human organ, and that potential shows up in various kinds of historical evidence. In 1998 a 5,400-year-old Egyptian mummy was found with a curved back that likely indicates the form of TB called Pott's disease. The DNA was amplified from the mummy and is similar to the current mycobacterium-complex. During the Middle Ages tuberculosis commonly showed up as inflamed and disfiguring bumps on the neck, a condition called scrofula.

Then the world discovered the Industrial Revolution. This promoted the rise of cities and increased air pollution, and TB moved into people's lungs on a much wider scale. The foul air that spewed from England's great factories of the early 1800s damaged human lungs so much that mycobacteria found a new favourite host. In the 1850s, when Americans visited England to see the wonders of industry, many were more impressed by the choking smog and stinking rivers. Anyone who has visited China in the last decade will not be surprised that the Chinese have a giant problem with pulmonary TB: you can't sit down on an outdoor bench in a major city without wiping the coal dust off first, a good clue to what you're breathing.

TREATING TB IN THE OLD DAYS

Doctors love to classify and name diseases, and with TB there was a plethora of names for the disease before the actual pathogen was discovered: it was called pthisis, consumption, white plague, the wasting disease, and so on. But in 1839 a professor of medicine in Zurich, J.L. Schönlein, suggested the word "tuberculosis" should be used as a single name for all versions of phthisis, since the tubercle was common to them all. Tubercles and tuberculous cavities in the lungs were discovered before the bacillus that caused the disease because doctors were performing autopsies on people who died of TB. Italian doctors in the 16th century already believed that TB was contagious. In order to do diagnostic work on a live patient, an 18th century Austrian physician named Leopold Auenbrugger invented "percussion," where a doctor taps on the patient's chest and makes a diagnosis based on the sound. This work was made easier with René Laënnec's invention of the stethoscope early in the 19th century.

In 1865 Jean Antoine Villemin, a French army surgeon, used experiments on animals to establish that TB was contagious. He injected rabbits with tuberculous material from cattle and from humans. By a cruel twist of fate, his work with this dangerous material infected him and he died of tuberculosis in 1892. Because he was only an army surgeon, though, he was not taken seriously as a scientist.

It was a German doctor, Robert Koch, who established in 1882 that TB is an infectious disease caused by a bacterium. Within days of Koch's discovery he was famous – the telegraph wires, the 19th century equivalent of CNN, were humming with the news. It took a mere three weeks for Koch to publish his discovery in a Berlin medical journal. By then everyone knew. He was both innovative and technically methodical in his laboratory work, and pioneered ways to dry and stain bacteria for examination under the microscope and ways to grow bacteria in culture that are used to this day. Koch also invented what he thought was a vaccine against TB that was later used as a substance for skin-testing in TB diagnosis. A version of this substance is used to this day for performing TB skin tests.

When William Konrad Roentgen discovered the x-ray in 1895, for which he won the first Nobel Prize in physics, the foundations of modern TB diagnostics were laid. Sputum samples from patients could be examined under the microscope and cultured for drug testing, skin tests could be given to suspected cases, and x-rays could take pictures of the lungs so that doctors would no longer depend on difficult guess-work with a stethoscope.

During the 19th and early 20th centuries TB killed about a billion people. Disease rates flared up again during the world wars. Doctors started their own all-out war on TB that included surgery, vaccines, numerous x-rays, and lengthy stays in sanatoria. None of these measures were particularly effective, although they certainly made the average person extremely aware of the dangers of TB, including the dangers of medical treatment.

As we've already seen, Germany and Switzerland pioneered the TB sanatorium, where patients went on extended and micromanaged bed rest over-seen by doctors. The sanatoria were a rallying point for efforts against the white death, a symbol of successful fundraising and the march of medical progress. But reality was uncooperative. A study published in the *American Review of Tuberculosis* in 1922, for example, showed that for nine sanatoria for which good statistics were available, 51% of the discharged patients were dead within five years. Perhaps the best thing that can be said about the sanatoria is that they isolated the most infectious TB patients and thus prevented them from spreading the disease to others. For the majority of patients, though, the benefits were often dubious.

One of the benefits of sanatorium stays was supposed to be lung surgery. Collapse therapy, along with removal or resection were the two major categories of surgery for TB treatment. Resection involved removing a diseased part of the lung, much as a tumour is removed from cancer patients today. Collapse therapy involved forcing one or both lobes of the lung to rest through a variety of surgical techniques.

TB doctors through the first half of the 20th century refused to simply provide palliative care and let people die in peace. Instead, they started performing a lot of invasive surgeries, some of which were, according to modern experts, worse than doing nothing. Most of their ideas revolved around the mistaken notion of resting the diseased lung. Doctors had noticed that patients who had a lot of bed rest appeared more likely to survive their TB. Before judging this belief or the eagerness with which doctors performed drastic surgery, it must be remembered that the modern idea of the clinical trial wasn't invented until about 1950. Michael Iseman of the National Jewish Center in Denver says that

We don't really know a lot about TB surgery's effectiveness before 1950 because the method of cohort analysis didn't exist in that era. You'd see a report saying 'we operated on 25 patients and 15 of them got well,' but we have no idea how they were selected, or what would have happened to them otherwise, so by conventional criteria there were no systematic data to guide us.

In other words no one methodically compared patient outcomes in a group of patients who got bed rest or surgery with a group who were not treated that way. Instead, doctors practised based on anecdotal evidence. As Iseman puts it:

There was lore, and the lore of surgery before drugs was that it was very hazardous. If you opened the ribs and cut out part of the lungs in the old days the patients did terribly because if you cut through active tuberculosis the wound would infect and patients often had very complicated miserable deaths. So instead of re-sectional surgery what was done was a variety of efforts to collapse the lung and close the cavities within the lung.

Lung resection surgery is still used on TB patients, but only very rarely, in combination with drug therapy, and in cases where the patient is likely to die without this intervention. Michael Iseman and his team at the National Jewish Center in Denver do still perform some of these surgical procedures, but only on patients who have drug resistant TB that cannot be completely cured with drugs. The National Jewish Center receives referrals of difficult TB cases from all over the United States. When Iseman arrived in 1982, only two-thirds of patients with drug resistant TB were being cured, "a dismal rate." The other third either died of TB or were pariahs since they were infectious and no one could be around them. So Iseman decided to revive TB surgery. After they started doing surgery on TB patients, cure rates rose from 56% to 85%, and total death rates fell dramatically as well. The program also saved money – even with the high cost of chest surgery, the net cost was lower because hospital stays were much shorter.

Iseman describes collapse therapy, which is now obsolete, like this:

What you would do is let air into the chest space to compress the lung, which is called pneumothorax, or re-shape the ribs to collapse the lung, called thoracoplasty, and then they also did "plombage" where they put Lucite balls within the chest or paraffin in it to compress the lung.

The sanatoria that sprung up all over the world, including Manitoba, typically had surgical facilities and performed a lot of surgery on TB patients. Starting in the 1920s it was common to induce what was called "artificial pneumothorax," which involved patients getting a painful injection of air into their chest to keep the lung from filling up and functioning normally. Often even outpatients would have to return frequently to the sanatorium to get their "pneumothorax refills."

The most brutal and invasive surgery was called thoracoplasty. This involved the removal of the ribs on one side to permanently collapse the diseased part of a lung. Thoracoplasty meant the chest area looked like it had been crushed, although at the time surgeons claimed no one would notice when the patient was clothed.

Iseman says that it is difficult for younger doctors to understand that as recently as the 1940s patients had a 60% chance of dying within five years from TB, so it wasn't surprising that surgeons tried radical procedures. This is what he says lung resection was like:

> If you cut through a bronchus to remove the right upper lobe and you had no antibiotics to suppress the TB, the surgeon would try to close off that bronchus but the bronchial closure wouldn't hold, so the bronchus would open and the TB would infect the chest wall where the patient's surgery had been closed and it would break through the chest wall. All of those nightmarish stories drove people away from surgery.

When Iseman's team started doing TB surgery again in the 1980s at National Jewish Hospital, they had "the advantage of being able to get a good enough antibiotic regimen that we could make surgery safe." The regimen did not always cure the patient, but it reduced the risks of surgery.

Dr. Peter Warren, of the University of Manitoba, says that we need to remember that medicine is about reducing suffering, not necessarily about curing disease. While we always hope that disease can be cured, the fact is that not even the wonder drugs of the 20th century, or gene-sequencing, or advanced micro-surgical techniques, or any of a dozen other technological advances, will guarantee the eradication of any disease. In the end, doctors and patients need to accept that sometimes all we can do is lessen the suffering involved in our inevitable mortality.

MODERN TB TREATMENT

Selman Waksman, along with two graduate assistants, discovered streptomycin, the first effective drug treatment for tuberculosis in 1943. Waksman was a Russian immigrant and a soil microbiologist who knew very little about disease pathology – he was not a doctor. Waksman did his work at the Rutgers Agricultural College in New Jersey and by 1943 was collaborating with doctors from the Mayo Clinic in Rochester, Minnesota. "Patricia T.", a young Minnesotan woman with severe TB, was actually the second TB patient to get streptomycin, and the first to be successfully treated. She was admitted to a sanatorium in

Cannon Falls, Minnesota in 1943. By 1944 she was desperately ill, so with nothing left to lose, her doctors gave her streptomycin. She made a full recovery and bore three healthy children in the 1950s, and then lived into old age. Merck and Company had already signed on to manufacture the new drug. An effective treatment for TB had finally been found. As Earl Hershfield puts it, "Patricia T. was lucky, and the whole TB world was lucky that she responded to streptomycin."

Streptomycin is also important in the history of medicine because of its association with the modern controlled drug trial. In 1948, the British Medical Research Council published what would be the seminal paper for clinical drug trials, a paper that also established the efficacy of streptomycin in treating TB.

However, nothing was ever simple or easy with tuberculosis. There were problems with side-effects from the drug, and with finding correct dosages. George Wherrett, whose book *The Miracle of the Empty Beds* is the definitive history of TB in Canada for its time (1977), is unusually frank about drug side-effects. He says that streptomycin's toxic effects included "damage to the VIIIth cranial nerve, causing dizziness, loss of balance, and deafness." Other drugs were needed.

European researchers continued working through the war years and afterwards to develop new drugs to fight disease. In the 1930s and '40s German pharmaceutical companies developed the drug para-aminosalicylic acid, or PAS. While this drug killed the TB bacillus, it was also very toxic to humans. Then Bayer, in Germany, and Squibb and Hoffman-La Roche in the US found isoniazid, or INH. In the fall of 1951, doctors at the Sea View Hospital, a TB sanatorium in New York, gave advanced TB patients the new drug. *Life* magazine published a picture of patients treated with INH dancing in the halls of Sea View Hospital.

INH was an extraordinary success and reamins part of the standard drug regimen for TB. It was well-tolerated and inexpensive, and INH was soon the centre-piece of TB treatment. There was early recognition that drug resistance could emerge if patients were treated with only one or two medications, so other drugs were used in combination with INH. PAS was often used, but it was hard on patients, and a new drug, ethambutol, was expensive. However, since ethambutol had fewer side effects, it soon replaced PAS.

Rarely has medical treatment for a disease changed so rapidly. Within five years of the introduction of drug therapy for TB, rest therapy had become a subject for medical history textbooks. Of course that did not mean that medical practice changed instantly all over the world. In Manitoba, as in many places, change would be linked to the retirement of key doctors who ran established TB institutions. Another hugely important factor would be the entry of younger doctors like Earl Hershfield, who was just coming out of medical training that included two years at the very Mayo Clinic where the modern TB treatment era began.

The standard treatment for TB is currently a four-drug cocktail taken over a six to nine month period. It's called RIPE, and it stands for the four drugs most effective against standard TB: Rifampin, Isoniazid, Pyrazinamide, and Ethambutol. Often these drugs are combined into a single pill to make the drugs easier to take. Rifampin, the youngest of these drugs, came on the market more than 30 years ago.

In the last five decades there has been very little in the way of new drugs or new diagnostics for tuberculosis. One of the few developments has been the approval of rifapentine as a so-called orphan drug in 1998. An "orphan drug" is a special regulatory category for a drug that treats a disease so rare that there is no financial incentive for the pharmaceutical company to bring the drug to market. With millions of people dying every year of TB, that category would seem misplaced for a TB drug. However, the term orphan diseases is now used broadly to cover common diseases that affect mostly poor people in developing countries. The lack of new drug development is especially significant for these countries because drug resistance is most common in the developing world.

DRUG RESISTANCE

When you ask patients to take large quantities of pills that have serious side-effects, and do so for many months, it is not surprising that you have compliance problems. TB can mutate into drug resistant or multi-drug-resistant (MDR) forms if medications are misused. The most common form of misuse is failure to complete the lengthy TB drug regimen. Often patients feel better after a few weeks on medication and stop taking their pills before completing the six to nine month course of treatment that TB currently requires. In poor countries the drug supply sometimes simply runs out, or drugs are mis-prescribed. Sometimes patients live in isolated areas and cannot get their drugs. There has been resistance to TB drugs right from the beginning of the modern drug treatment era in the 1950s.

What is the mechanism that causes drug resistance when a patient, for any reason, takes an incomplete dosage of TB antibiotics? Joyce Wolfe of the national TB laboratory explains it this way: "How does the bug develop resistance? Say you have a million organisms in this one colony. In every colony there's a certain percentage that are intrinsically resistant to some of the drugs." If a patient stops treatment after taking only one drug, you don't get rid of the organisms that are sensitive only to other drugs and you end up with some of the resistant ones being untreated.

Think of these resistant TB germs as a colony of athletes in a village, and the village is usually the patient's lungs. The athletes that are intrinsically resistant to particular drugs, are stronger and more competitive than the others in the life-and-death struggle they are preparing for. The early stages of the drug treatment destroy the germs that are sensitive to whatever drug the patient takes. Now the stronger, more competitive germs reproduce. If the drug treatment is cut off early, what happens is that the patient is actually encouraging a selection process that allows some bugs to survive and reproduce, becoming tougher in the process. These new mutant TB germs include genetic information that makes them resistant to some of the standard "first-line" drugs used to treat TB – potentially anything in the four-drug cocktail called RIPE. Further treatments with some of these first-line drugs can actually make the patient worse once drug resistance sets in.

Much of the drug resistance in the developing world is caused not only by incomplete treatments, but also by improper use of TB drugs. Russian doctors are notorious for making up their own cocktails of TB drugs and vitamins and prescribing them in arbitrary dosages, a surefire recipe for creating drug resistance. John Sbarbaro, a professor of medicine at the University of Colorado, told me that "in countries like the Philippines and Indonesia, TB drugs are available over the counter and pharmacists make up bags of vitamins and isoniazid or rifampin as cough medicine." A high degree of government cooperation is essential in preventing inappropriate use of medicine.

The World Health Organization's technical definition of multi-drug-resistant (MDR) TB goes like this: it is TB resistant to the two most important anti-TB drugs, isoniazid and rifampin. According to World Health Organization figures, over 50 million people may be infected with drug-resistant strains of the disease. MDR TB is not a death sentence, but it is harder and more expensive to treat than regular TB. In other words it is a death sentence for the majority of its victims, since these people live mostly in poor countries that lack good health care systems. Patients with MDR TB have to take drugs for up to 24 months, instead of a mere six to nine months. The second-line drugs that they need are considerably more expensive than the standard ones, often by a factor of 100 times. Cure rates go down from about 95% to as little as 50%, and that's when treatment is actually available. Of course the numbers are worse where people are poor. This is because of the added cost for the drugs, the long time that people have to take them for, and the sophisticated lab work that is usually needed to correctly treat an MDR case. The typical procedure is to take a coughed-up sputum sample from a patient and test it with various TB drugs to find out which drugs it is resistant or sensitive to. Because the TB germ or bacillus grows very slowly, it will take weeks to get the results back. Of course this presumes the existence of a high tech laboratory with well-trained technicians, when the reality is that many countries can't even provide their labs with reliable electricity or refrigerators.

DOTS: THE BIG ACRONYM IN TB CONTROL

"THE BIGGEST PROBLEM WITH THIS DISEASE IS THAT PATIENTS
DON'T TAKE THEIR MEDS."
— EARL HERSHFIELD

The solution to getting TB under control is, at the most superficial level, to make drug treatment available to everyone who has the disease. However, that's not enough. Side-effects of just one of the four standard TB drugs, for example, can include nausea and vomiting, joint aches, rashes, fevers, and fatigue. Research shows that only half of patients will complete their drug regimen if left on their own. How do you ensure that people take the full course of medication?

The answer is the international standard for TB control, adopted by the World Health Organization (the WHO) and more than 120 countries: Directly Observed Therapy, Short-course, or DOTS. DOTS was originally developed by the International Union Against Tuberculosis and Lung Disease (IUATLD) and the WHO adopted it in the late 1990s. DOTS as a treatment standard involves three elements: health care workers directly observing patients taking their medicine, a TB reporting system that tracks cases and contacts, and free treatment to patients. DOTS is an outpatient model, so instead of expensive stays in the hospital and lengthy disruption of patients' lives, treatment is delivered directly to patients where they live or in an easily accessed clinic.

Although directly observed therapy, which was sometimes also called case management and directly administered therapy, has really been around since the 1970s, it only became the global standard in the 1990s. Previously it was often reserved for only problematic cases, and still is sometimes when resources are limited. Many studies have shown that compliance with the lengthy drug regimens typical of TB treatment go from about 50% to above 95% when DOTS is used. DOTS prevents patients from stopping their treatment before they have had the full course of medication, and this prevents the almost inevitable relapses of the disease. Relapses, or reactivations as doctors call them, are much harder to treat since the patients are now likely to be drug resistant.

A Hungarian doctor named Karol Styblo, more than anyone else, did the epidemiological work that made DOT the world standard for treating TB. Styblo worked for the Royal Netherlands TB Association and the IUATLD for many years, including pioneering work on DOTS in Tanzania. He died in 1998. The World Bank now considers DOT to be the equivalent of a vaccine against TB, and while that is over-optimistic it shows the profound importance of Styblo's work. Styblo himself got TB in a Nazi concentration camp in 1945. Earl Hershfield describes Styblo as "a very big influence on my life" and "one of the best TB epidemiologists in the world."

There were at least two elements of Styblo's strategy that broke new ground. First, he advocated "short-course chemotherapy," which was drug treatment for only six to eight months, and he advocated using it in developing countries. This cut treatment times in half and encouraged patients to complete their treatment. Second, Styblo's recording and reporting system was new. Health workers were accountable for observing and recording patients taking their meds. You no longer needed to hospitalise most TB patients during their whole treatment period.

Many health officials in the 1970s were sitting on their hands. They thought that TB could not be controlled in poor countries until socio-economic conditions improved. Styblo disagreed, stubbornly and strongly. His tenacity showed in the results he got, doubling cure rates in countries like Tanzania and in a pilot project in China in the early 1990s that involved about two million people. Earl travelled with Styblo all over Asia in the 1980s, setting up treatment programs like the ones he began in Africa.

There were other pioneers of DOT too. John Sbarbaro was the very young medical officer of health in Denver by 1966, and he implemented DOT, spurred by reading journals and ignoring the consternation of older colleagues. His employers in government were delighted. Not only did cure rates go up, but costs went down drastically as he emptied the TB ward in the local hospital. Sbarbaro used quarantine orders when necessary to ensure that patients came back to get their meds, and he gave them intensive drug therapy in hospital for only two to three months. This is exactly the model that is used by contemporary TB control programs in North America.

In Manitoba, as in many other parts of the world, family physicians were not always enthusiastic about directly observed therapy. It seemed silly to them that someone would have to literally watch a patient taking medicine and then record that it took place. Doctors complained that patients would feel they weren't trusted if they had to be observed taking pills. Nurses didn't always like the idea of having community health workers dispensing pills either – after all what would nurses do if they weren't giving pills to patients? Interestingly, similar issues arise in many places where DOT is introduced. For example, in Russia, many doctors are opposed to DOT, which they see as something that's only appropriate in developing countries. They are often extremely reluctant to let non-doctors give out pills. Many Russian doctors now are behaving like North American doctors did in the sanatorium era before 1950, when it was common for a doctor to customize and then micro-manage a "rest therapy" for each patient. What's worse is that many Russian doctors customize drug regimens for TB patients, which leads directly to drug resistance and disease that is more difficult to deal with.

The standardization of treatment in DOTS has in itself led to some problems with drug resistant TB. Originally the standard treatment was to repeat a six month round of the common four-drug cocktail if the patient was not cured by the first go-round. However, Dr. Paul Farmer and his colleagues in Haiti and Peru discovered that these stubborn cases needed to be treated differently. Because drug resistant cases are actually unique, here customized combinations of drugs are appropriate — these combinations consist of second-line TB drugs chosen on the basis of laboratory analysis of the patient's sputum, however, not arbitrarily selected by a doctor without laboratory support. As a result of Farmer's work, the WHO now has a special protocol called DOTS Plus for the treatment of drug resistant TB that provides guidelines for the customized treatment needed for MDR TB. They also have a "Green Light Committee" that monitors and approves second-line drugs for drug resistant TB programs, to ensure that the drugs are used properly.

One nurse in Manitoba told me a story about how she had to educate an intern who was trying to prescribe drugs for a TB patient living up north. The intern had prescribed drugs that needed to be injected, which meant that the patient would have to come in to a nursing station for treatment. The nurse pointed out that this wasn't practical because the patient lived in an isolated community, far from any nursing station. Judgement needs to be exercised, even with a standardized regimen; patients need medicines appropriate to their situations, and monitoring by community health workers also needs to make sense for the situation.

Sometimes extraordinary measures need to be taken to break the cycle that is typical for people who have TB – a cycle where poor people are sick, and sick people are poor. In other words it may be that patients fail to take their medications, but health systems need to be adaptive so that they understand why patients behave the way they do. Examples of this often arise in developing countries. Research has shown that patients will not walk more than about nine kilometres to get treatment. What if the clinic is more than nine kilometres away? What if the clinic runs out of drugs before the treatment period is complete? What if there are no technicians who can prepare slides and read sputum samples with microscopes? What if there are no refrigerators to store the cultures, and no reliable electricity for the fridges? And of course if there is not even reliable census data, how can a country be expected to have accurate reporting of TB, which is an essential part of a control system?

In addition, it is absolutely essential that governments and politicians support efforts to control disease. There are no charitable or nongovernmental organizations that can solve a country's whole TB problem. Ultimately the government must do it. However, if a government is preoccupied with a structural adjustment program imposed on it by the World Bank, then privatising the water supply so a multinational corporation can make more money for their shareholders may be a bigger priority than public health.

One of the key benefits of DOTS, as the World Bank has recognized since 1993, is exactly its cost effectiveness, largely because the directly observed therapy model makes extensive use of community healthcare workers. Unfortunately, as of

2001, only 33% of the world's TB cases had access to DOTS treatment. The United Nation's Millenium Development Goals for health will never be reached with such a low level of access to DOTS; the millennium goal for TB is that the disease prevalence and death rates should be halved by 2015.

VACCINATION FOR TB

DOTS itself as a strategy is a response to inadequate tools with which to attack TB. If a one-shot vaccine could be developed, like the one that eradicated smallpox, then there would be much less of a need for extended drug treatments. The only vaccine that exists today, BCG (Bacille Calmette-Guérin), is a live freeze-dried vaccine originally introduced in France in 1921, and its effectiveness is highly questionable. Globally, almost 85% of the world's children have been immunized against TB with BCG. The vaccine appears to provide protection against the most serious forms of childhood tuberculosis: miliary tuberculosis (which mainly affects the lungs but also spreads via the blood throughout the body) and tuberculous meningitis (which affects brain and spine). However, the vaccine's effectiveness against these forms of childhood TB is highly variable – somewhere between 50% and 80%. BCG offers some protection against leprosy, TB's mycobacterial cousin, but its protection against adult forms of tuberculosis is uncertain at best. BCG also complicates skin testing by producing false positives.

The unpredictability of BCG is caused by the way it's prepared. John Sbarbaro explains the scientific problem like this:

> In the 1920s you took a bovine TB culture, grew it, and then moved it from one culture plate to the next one every 6 weeks, because that's how long it takes to get 72 million bugs, enough to make a culture. Then you have to make it less virulent by re-culturing it many times so you got a weaker bovine TB. You gave it to kids. How did you know it worked? Because you studied how many people who were immunized got TB ten years later. Then you said, 'OK, we've got a good vaccine. Let's go back and get a sample of that.' Trouble is that for the eight years in-between, you're still growing it every six weeks. So you go back and take a sample out of that existing BCG. How do you know you didn't get a stronger or weaker one? Sometimes you got a stronger one and it killed people, sometimes you got a weaker one that had no impact. Then we decided to freeze the product in the '70s. You made one big batch of the vaccine, you froze it, you gave it to people, and guess what? We froze a wimp. It didn't give any protection. This doesn't mean that earlier vaccines didn't give protection, it means that the only product we actually had hard core data on turned out to be worthless.

Ultimately the world needs both a therapeutic vaccine for people who already have TB, and a prophylactic vaccine to prevent getting the disease; having both of these in one syringe would be ideal. Research is under way to develop a new vaccine that would be more effective in preventing childhood TB and maybe even extend protection into early adulthood when most adult cases occur. Much of this research activity can be attributed to the outbreak of TB in the US in the late 1980s. Whatever the cause, the world desperately needs a more effective TB vaccine.

Even Dr. George Comstock, a world-famous TB epidemiologist who has spent his whole career advocating against the widespread use of BCG in the US, told me that if he ran a TB program in the developing world he would use BCG. He says the vaccine is tremendously cheap, valuable healthcare infrastructure is built up with vaccination programs, and it has a good chance of preventing childhood forms of TB. The World Health Organization similarly recommends that all countries with a high incidence of TB infection should immunize children under five with a single dose of BCG. Booster doses of BCG are not recommended by the World Health Organization and only a few countries, like Russia, continue to use them.

HIV/AIDS: THE DEADLIEST ACRONYM

If you think of TB as a product for sale all over the world, you would have to conclude that while the product has not changed much at all, the opportunity to sell the product has improved recently in an at least one dramatic way. That is co-infection of TB with HIV/AIDS.

If we were going to put our metaphorical TB germ/athletes from the earlier discussion of drug resistance on steroids, there is nothing that would make them stronger than the human immunovirus or HIV infection. TB and the HIV infection together actually speed up each other's progress. TB is an opportunistic infection, and AIDS is the big jackpot for tuberculosis. In Africa, about one third of the people who die with HIV infection actually die of TB – HIV and AIDS just soften them up by destroying their immune systems. People who have HIV are about 480 times more likely to have their latent TB infection activated. By the early 1990s, most adults in sub-Saharan Africa, Haiti, and Asia, already had latent TB infection. Unless TB is controlled in these populations, there's not a chance that HIV will be. All over the world health care professionals are increasingly worried about the deadly co-infection of HIV and TB. The prospect of that co-infection being between HIV and multi-drug-resistant TB is even more frightening.

MDR TB is a serious problem in countries like Haiti, where a larger percentage of the adult population is HIV positive. In Russia, MDR TB is especially common in the gigantic prison system, which turns over 300,000 people every year. Of these, 10% have active, infectious TB, and probably a third of those have MDR TB. Because Russia is just beginning to see larger numbers of HIV cases, largely because of intravenous drug use, this will be a new tinderbox of disease. Why should those of us who live in wealthy countries with excellent health care systems care? Lee Reichman answers this question in two words: "people travel." In a world of cheap and constant air travel, disease will travel along with people, especially a disease that you get by breathing.

WHY TB IS COMING BACK EVERYWHERE

While the global HIV pandemic and multi-drug-resistant strains of TB are both contributing to the spread of TB, these two causes are not the whole story. Global travel, homelessness, and the increasing number of refugees moving around because of war is also helping to spread the germs. An intercontinental flight in a pressurized cabin from Russia to New York, for example, could be a perfect opportunity for someone to catch TB. You only need to be around someone who's coughing and infectious for about eight hours to have a chance to catch TB.

In terms of refugees and displaced people there are many who will and should be admitted to countries like Canada. Because refugees are constantly on the move it is hard to treat them with the current six month drug regimen. Citizenship and Immigration Canada have a protocol to deal with screening refugees for TB and doing follow-up treatment with those who have latent disease, but the fact is that TB cannot be dismissed as someone else's problem. No one can stop international travel and trade.

The New York press was full of headlines in the early 1990s about an outbreak of drug-resistant TB that started in jails. The fact that the victims were jail guards and not merely prisoners was what grabbed people's attention. New York eventually spent $1 billion fighting 4,000 cases. Much of the money went into health care infrastructure that was dismantled back when it looked like TB had been eradicated in the US, exactly when public health experts like Lee Reichman were predicting that TB would come back. The Canadian numbers started to climb again in 1989, near the time of the New York epidemic. Right now London, England is the TB capital of the world, with double the level of New York's case-load in the 1990s. Even though England is a rich country, homeless people live on London's streets in conditions just as squalid as anything George Orwell wrote about in the 1930s. Disease does not respect boundaries or wealth. But without wealth no one can fight disease.

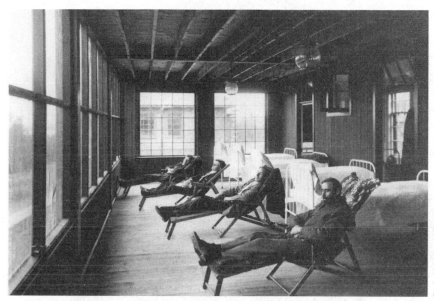

Patients taking the rest cure for TB, Manitoba Sanatorium at Ninette, interior of men's sleeping pavilion, about 1910.

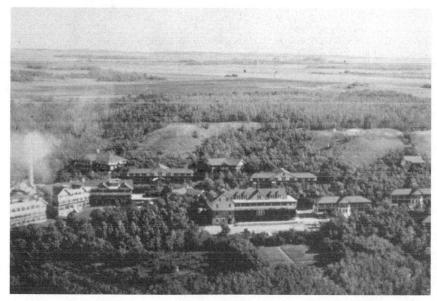

Aerial view of the Manitoba Sanatorium at Ninette, 1930. On the left are the east and west infirmaries with the powerhouse behind them. The nurses' residence is in the upper left with two "pavilions" for patients to the right. In the centre is the infirmary building with the Gordon cottage, main buildings, and women's observation pavilion to the right. At its peak the Sanatorium had 24 buildings.

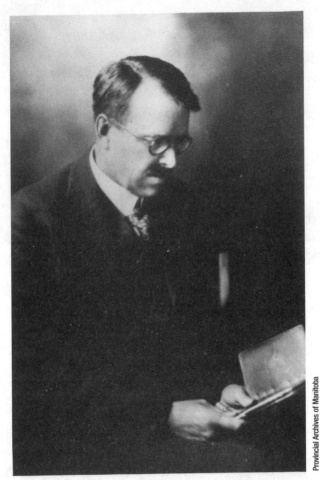

Provincial Archives of Manitoba

David A. Stewart, medical superintendent at Ninette Sanatorium from 1909 to 1937.

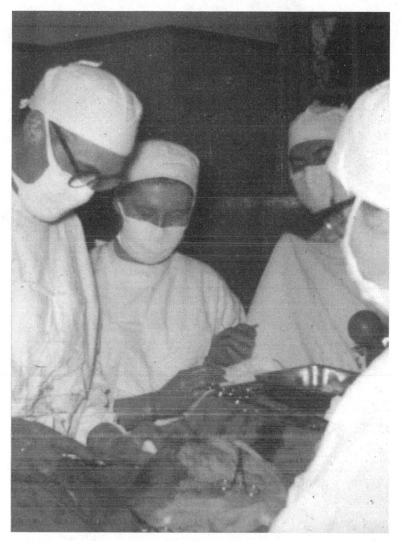

Western Canada Pictorial Index

A lung resection surgery in the operating room at Ninette, 1955. Presiding are Dr. A.L. Paine, nurse Mary Blatz (OR supervisor), and Dr. M. Wasylzajcew (left to right).

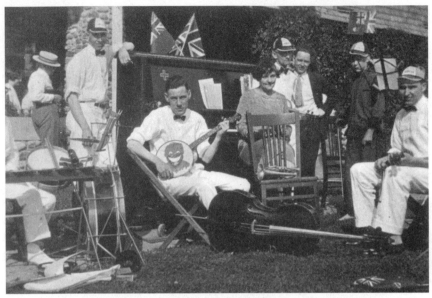

Ninette Sanatorium orchestra on July 1, 1927. David B. Stewart is second from right, age 10.

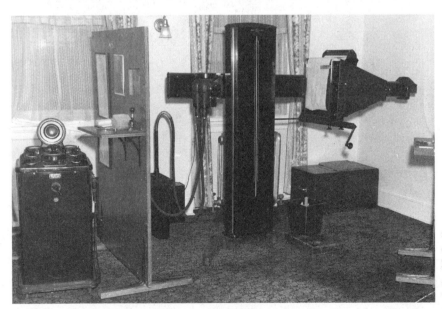

X-ray machine operated by the Sanatorium Board of Manitoba, ca. 1950s.

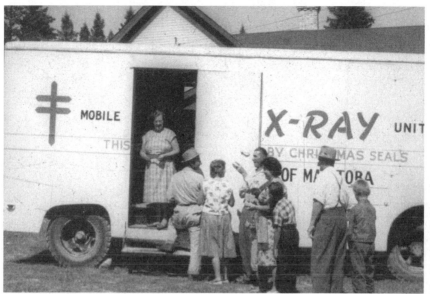

A mobile x-ray unit operated by the Sanatorium Board of Manitoba, 1963. These trucks traveled to every community in the province to screen for TB.

Western Canada Pictorial Index

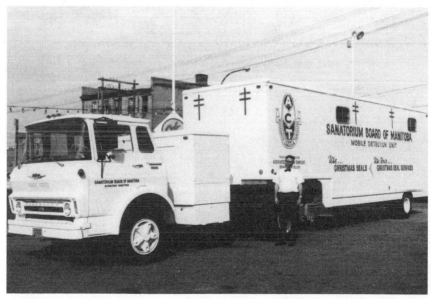

A mobile x-ray unit operated by the Sanatorium Board around 1970. Note the electrical generator to the right of the cab.

collection of Jim Zayshley

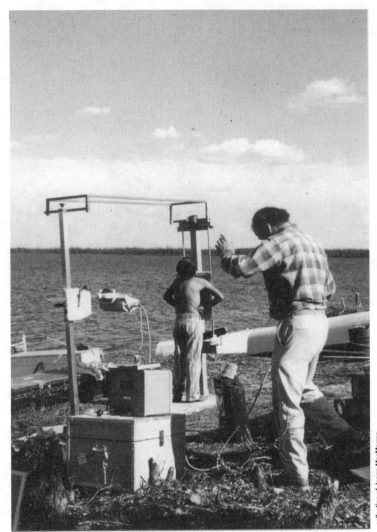

Earl Hershfield doing an x-ray at North Knife Lake, Manitoba, 1968.

collection of Joann MacMorran

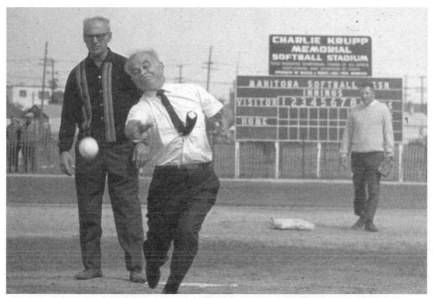

Earl's father, Sheppy Hershfield, former YMHA pitcher, throwing the first pitch at the opening of Charlie Krupp stadium in Winnipeg, 1967. His brother Leible and Terry O'Sipa (right) look on.

Western Canada Pictorial Index

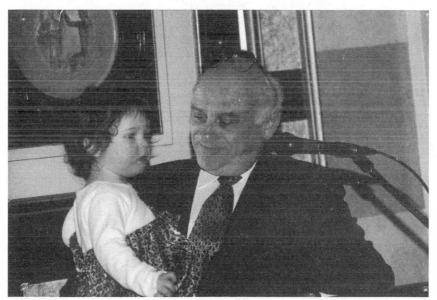

Earl Hershfield with his granddaughter Sophia Hershfield, at the 90th birthday of Earl's mother, Teenie, 2000.

Manuel F. Sousa Photography

Service of Remembrance

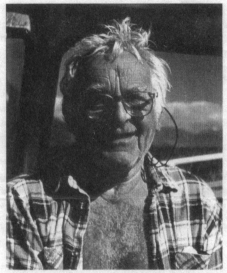

collection of Anne Fanning

STEFAN GRZYBOWSKI

b.   January 13, 1920,   Warsaw, Poland
d.   September 9, 1997, Vancouver, Canada

Carpe Diem

Funeral program for Stefan Grzybowski, pioneering Canadian TB researcher and doctor.

5

MAIN STREET AND THE LIVING DISEASE

"I'VE BEEN FIGHTING LIKE A LION, LOOKS LIKE
I'M GOIN' TO LOSE....I'VE GOT THE TB BLUES."
— JIMMY ROGERS, "TB BLUES"

All over North America in the early 1990s TB was making a comeback, especially among people living on the street. In Winnipeg there was a serious outbreak of TB between 1990 and 1994 on the Main Street strip of seedy hotels and shelters for the homeless. There were more than 100 people with active TB on the strip in those years, a staggering increase from the normal handful of cases that anyone in TB control would have expected. Dr. Lawrence Elliott, now director of the Community Medicine Residency Program at the University of Manitoba, wrote his master's thesis on this TB outbreak. One of his thesis advisors was Earl Hershfield, who together with Joann MacMorran, were the pivotal figures in controlling the outbreak – Earl in his role as Medical Director and Joann as Nurse Consultant, co-ordinating the contact investigations. Elliott describes their work as "innovative," because what they did was take TB screening and treatment out to the homeless population of the Main Street area. They did not expect that street people would suddenly start going to hospitals or clinics. Instead they had workers at shelters dispense TB medications and at some points even had bartenders at Main Street hotels doing directly observed therapy with their clientele.

Among the 100 active TB cases, many were clients of the Main Street Project, a shelter for street people in the area. Elliott's investigation proved what Earl and Joann already suspected, which was that many of the cases had contracted the disease from each other while sleeping in an overcrowded room at the Main Street Project. Earl recommended a larger space for the Main Street Project's clients to sleep in, and an improved ventilation system. By 1994 there were once again only a handful of TB cases in the area, but the Main Street Project had implemented Earl's recommendations and maintains x-ray equipment on-site to this day. Every few months the Manitoba Lung Association's team comes in and takes chest x-rays of both clients and staff.

Elliott remembers that a single TB case in a public school garnered more attention with the Winnipeg media than the entire outbreak of the early 1990s. This chapter tells the story of how TB went from being a disease that affected everyone, including the middle class and even the famous, to one that primarily affects those who are socially marginalized.

DONUTS AND X-RAYS

It's 6:45 am in December 2003, on the front steps of the Main Street Project in downtown Winnipeg. The day outside is cold, but not what a Winnipegger would call really cold. About 20 people form a tight group on the steps, some laughing, some bleary-eyed, all of them looking like they slept in their clothes. The clothes appear to be the result of random acts of charity or scrounging. A skinny man with a purple hoody and a laser pointer stares into space and then at everyone else, with the laser pointer dancing around. Two of the men in line are white, all the others are Aboriginal; there are only a couple of women. One of the white guys has an orange Bacardi gym bag slung on his shoulder. The other one is built like a linebacker and carries three bags, with an insulated vest instead of a coat. One person has a scarf wrapped around his head. There's a woman in a bright blue and orange snow suit. One guy has a Marathon airlines cap, another an Aero gym bag.

"Hey they're takin' x-rays this morning," somebody says loudly when the door opens for a minute to allow only six people in. The worker at the door, who's holding a walkie-talkie, says they won't get their coffee and donuts until they have an x-ray. The white linebacker says "fuck this" and stomps off into the north wind. He's back within half an hour. The survey team from the Manitoba Lung Association can process about 40 people per hour with a crew of three. This morning they will give 58 people x-rays. The worker at the door talks on his walkie to someone inside who monitors the line at the x-ray machine. Still, no one is used to this delay in getting breakfast. One guy moons the others in line, pulling down his over-size bright green polyester track pants. There is a lot of back-slapping. Many of the men have dirty bandages wrapped around their hands, as if they often have close encounters with glass or knives.

Inside the Main Street Project there's one line to get x-rays, and then another one for donuts and coffee. The antique-looking x-ray machine has its own narrow room. At the end of the room is the business end of the x-ray. This is a cathode tube that projects the x-ray mounted on a column, and attached to the column is a control panel that maybe came out of *20,000 Leagues Under the Sea*. Behind the control panel is a small curtained area with a box for the x-ray films. At the other end of the room the patients turn their backs to the column with the x-ray and stand against the wall, where there are two sliding rails that hold the film in a metal cassette. Inside this wall is a lead lining to protect the office on the other side. This is a permanent installation – it came from a hospital where it was sitting in storage. When one technician measures the patient's chest with a set of calipers, he calls out the number ("21," "23") to the other tech at the control panel, and the other tech adjusts the intensity of the x-ray by turning a knob. Then the first tech says "take a deep breath and hold it." There is a thwock sound and then the tech at the panel says "OK. Next." The patient turns around, puts his coat back on, and shuffles out to the door, almost bumping into the next person.

Outside the x-ray room another tech sits at a small table, writing names and addresses down on a yellow form with a tear-off piece that has information about TB. When the tech says "address?" a lot of people laugh. "How 'bout here?" Sometimes he asks where they usually go and they give him the names of soup kitchens, bars, and hotels around Main Street. The tech fills in treaty numbers for Aboriginal people. The first three digits of the complete number, which denote the band number, don't usually get recorded; instead the tech writes the name of the band. The next 4 digits is what everybody gives – this is the individual number. The birth dates of the people in line today range from the late 1930s to the 1980s. Everyone looks at least a decade older than what they say. Many of the faces are pock-marked and puffy, with shadows of more distinct features that existed at some earlier point in their lives.

When the rush clears, the tech tells me a local legend. There was a guy who lived on the street and gave his address as the Main Street Project who won $100,000 in a lottery. No one saw him around the Project for a couple of months while he gave away all his money to his friends on the street, holding extensive symposia in Main Street bars until the money ran out. Then he was back at the Main Street Project.

The Main Street Project is a charitable organization that exists to help Winnipeg inner city adults who are homeless or not functioning well because of alcoholism or chemical dependency. About 65% of the clients have mental health problems as well as substance abuse issues. Quite a few are severely mentally ill. The public probably knows the Project best as a "drunk tank," or an "intoxicated persons detention area" in official parlance. The Winnipeg police fund the detention area on a fee-for-service basis. The agency operates a patrol that picks up individuals who are intoxicated after the bars close and brings them back for the night. The Main Street Project also operates an emergency overnight shelter and a detox centre, and conducts advocacy with other agencies on behalf of clients. In addition they provide 34 beds of transitional housing for up to a year for people who want to stop living on the street.

The largest area inside the Main Street Project's location on Martha Street serves as a drop-in centre by day and a sleeping area by night. As many as 60 people sleep on the floor on thin blue gym mats of the kind found in every elementary school in Canada. Early in the morning, staff rouse the sleepers and they stack the mats up and mop the floor. Then they are returned to the street, where in a few minutes they line up again for breakfast. Various companies donate two-day old donuts.

On the other side from where the line forms for x-rays is the detox area, separated by two glass walls with an office in-between. There is a sign on the first glass wall saying "No Weapons or weapon-like items, No alcohol, No violence," followed by a promise of police intervention if any of these rules are contravened. The brick walls around the edge of the room are a calm blue.

"When do we find out?" one of the men in line asks the tech outside the x-ray room.

"No news is good news. If something is wrong we let you know." The tech is wearing a leather baseball cap and a t-shirt with faded jeans.

"I had TB one time. Don't know how I got it," continues the man in line, gesturing broadly. "Then I took pills for a year" – he makes a scooping motion – "and they said I was healthy. I took care of myself then. Ate good, no drinkin'. They said the TB was dormant, and it wouldn' come back."

"Well you need to stay healthy," says the tech.

"I'm not doing so good on that now. But maybe someday. Maybe I will someday." Looking at him, that seems less likely than peace in the Middle East. He is missing all his front teeth, his face is battered, and there's a dark swelling beside one eye.

The next morning the line is shorter in front of the Main Street Project, because most of the regulars have gotten their x-rays and by-passed that line this morning. People are peering through a window at a clock that faces outwards, waiting for seven o'clock. Every minute or so the guy in front pounds at the door. There is an extroverted, very short Aboriginal woman at the back of the line. She cheerfully greets everyone by name. "Hi Ruth, Hi Wayne, Good morning Raymond."

The same beefy white guy from yesterday morning is here again, complaining. "I want my fuckin' soup," he says, then repeats himself. No one pays any attention, or points out that soup will not be served. The cheerful woman says "There's a dead pigeon in the back alley." Everyone laughs, although it's not clear to whom she's talking.

Another short woman is with her, and she says "My zipper is broke. Doesn't go up." Her happy companion says "Don't take it off by the river" – she pauses – "and lay down on it." There is general laughter. The broken zipper woman responds but without defensiveness, "there's no dirt on the back."

The laughter makes the first woman more expansive. "We need some police around here. You people are making yourselves *conspicuous*." She emphasizes the last word the way drunks do when they can't remember something, as if anything longer than a grunt is inherently funny – and yet she uses the word exactly right, over-pronouncing it slightly.

Inside the building once the door opens there is a rush to get in the coffee line. Anyone who didn't get their x-ray yesterday gets intercepted and sent to the Manitoba Lung Association survey team, who record their names and particulars on the yellow forms and send them to the back room for their x-rays.

Once people get their coffee a general malaise sets in. One man stretches out on the floor with his shirt and jacket rolling up over his exposed belly to sleep off whatever his night held. Another guy sits on the edge of a metal frame with his jacket for a seat. A skinny white guy who looks like a lost '70s rock star sits on a folding chair reading a paperback. He wears cowboy boots and has an air of stylishness. The only activity is two guys shaving at sinks in an open area just around the corner.

A man named Raymond approaches one of the x-ray techs. He wears dark glasses and carries a cane that he uses to navigate. His hair is slicked back and rides high in front in an attempt at a pompadour. Raymond looks like he's impersonating a blues legend. He has an amplifier on his throat so he can make himself heard. He pushes the button and asks for Paul, one of the Main Street Project workers. The tech explains he's here to do x-rays and is not with the Project. Raymond shuffles off in the direction of donuts and coffee.

CASE-FINDING

Al Harmacy has been the Survey Officer for the Manitoba Lung Association since 1981. It's his job to supervise a three-man team that takes chest x-rays and administers tuberculin skin tests for TB throughout Manitoba. The team is part of what are called contact investigations: when someone is diagnosed anywhere in the province with TB, a public health nurse interviews the patient and finds out who they have been in contact with. "In the Main Street area, people routinely drink with each other, and there's no way to separate them out," says Al. When the survey team visits the Main Street Project, they typically find between one and five infectious cases of tuberculosis. So that means someone needs to find out what soup kitchens, hotels, and communities the person has been in, and then the team needs to test people at all those locations.

A computerized TB registry is kept at the Health Sciences Centre's Respiratory Hospital in Winnipeg, and the new patient's information and contacts are entered into the database. What the nurses who run the registry are looking for is the "index case," which is the original case who infected a number of other people. Al Harmacy's team does the testing on people in areas targeted through interviews and any other information that comes from TB patients, social workers, doctors, or others. Tests are done on a regular basis at social service agencies like the Main Street Project, at the Main Street hotels in Winnipeg that cater to the vulnerable populations who simply can't afford decent accommodation, at soup kitchens around the core of the city, and often in First Nations communities or reserves in the north of the province. Many of these tests or surveys are triggered by information received from the TB Control Program based at the Health Sciences Centre. Part of the complicated responsibility of the TB Registry is keeping track of movement of TB patients between northern communities and Winnipeg, and also trying to trace those who do not complete their medical regimens, thus compromising their own health and potentially that of others.

Al Harmacy says that "the public doesn't have a perception of TB." He elaborates: outside certain immigrant and Aboriginal communities, people assume that TB is something that either never happens or is easily dealt with, and is after all somebody else's problem. "I don't think that the general public is even aware that we still do medical testing for TB, or TB surveys, or contact investigations for TB," says Al. He shrugs a little bit. "The perception is that TB doesn't exist, TB is a thing of the past, but if someone comes in with it from overseas they treat the person and that's it. But it's a lot more complicated than that. It's following up on all the people around them."

Al spent a number of months in Macedonia in the mid-1990s helping set up an x-ray survey program to control TB there. Like many war-affected areas Macedonia had problems with TB. The Manitoba Lung Association got involved partly because of the equipment that they have: it's unique in the world at this point to have x-ray equipment that can be easily dismantled and moved around, and still produce full-size x-rays that are easy for chest doctors to read. Al Harmacy helped set up a survey team and operate the Manitoba equipment until Macedonia was able to purchase their own suitable x-ray equipment.

Al was making a sales call to the Lung Association for a medical equipment supplier in 1981 when he was offered the job of running the survey team. He already had x-ray experience and training with Cancer Care Manitoba and the provincial government. The Manitoba Lung Association was looking for someone to replace Jim Zayshley, the first person who held the job and to some extent invented it, starting in 1954.

THE VANISHING TRUCKS

"When we lost the trucks we lost everything" — Jim Zayshley

Jim Zayshley was the first Survey Officer for the Manitoba Lung Association, which was still called the Sanatorium Board of Manitoba when he started in 1954. His job was to organize a TB prevention program that visited every municipality in the province on a two-year repeating basis. Like many first-generation employees in non-profit organizations, Jim was a kind of entrepreneur, defining his own job. Also like many people in TB prevention, he got involved because he had the disease. Dr. Tony Scott diagnosed him with TB in 1941 after he had volunteered for the Canadian Air Force and gotten a screening x-ray. Dr. Scott described it as "a very small infection." Jim spent about six months in the Manitoba Sanatorium at Ninette. He was treated with the then-current method of rest therapy and an enriched diet. While Jim recovered, he showed a lot of interest in the laboratory and the disease. This in itself wasn't unusual; through the mid-1950s about half the trainees hoping to become x-ray technicians were former TB patients.

What was unusual was Jim's ambition: he wanted to use the newer portable x-ray equipment to do mass surveys of everyone in the province to screen them for TB. When I talked to Jim in November 2003, he was 87 years old and still gifted with a clear mind. He said that he told Dr. Scott, "why don't we extend chest x-rays into the community?" Jim went on: "that was my policy: to start teaching people, children too, and in high schools about TB so they would know what to do." And screen them, test them, and teach them he did, first for about ten years for the City of Winnipeg Health Department, and then for almost three decades after the Sanatorium Board hired him in 1954.

Over the course of his 28-year career, Jim logged about 1.6 million kilometres working in every community in Manitoba. He wrote radio spots advertising "free chest x-rays" with urgent pleas to join the "fight to wipe out tuberculosis." Jim wrote letters to mayors, reeves, town councilors, managers, union bosses, and Indian agents, always asking permission to come in with one of his traveling clinics. Large employers like Eaton's would have all their employees x rayed to make sure they didn't have TB. That's how Jim met his wife, Dolly, at the old Eaton's building in Winnipeg.

From the 1950s until the mid-1970s, the Sanatorium Board's public image could be summed up by the large white trucks with the Lorraine cross that carried portable x-ray equipment, pamphlets, and, later, materials for tuberculin skin tests. Each truck pulled its own high voltage generator behind it, and appeared at high schools, community centres, agricultural fairs, churches, and later at shopping malls. Whenever anyone saw one of these trucks, they immediately thought of the ever-present danger of TB, of the Board, and probably of Christmas Seals as well. Just a few years before his retirement, Jim said to Arlene Jones, then the Manitoba Lung Association's Education Director, "When we lost the trucks we lost everything." What he meant was that TB was becoming invisible to most people. The Ninette San was long gone, as were all the other sanatoria. But an infectious disease that still affects people at the margins of your community remains dangerous.

By the 1980s when Jim retired, a lot of things had changed: first mass x-rays for the population were replaced mostly by tuberculin skin tests, then diabetic surveys and pulmonary function tests were added. With the smaller number of TB patients, the program shifted to include a silicosis detection program for miners and other industrial workers. Finally, TB contact follow-up mostly replaced mass testing campaigns.

Patrick Friesen, a distinguished Canadian poet who grew up in Steinbach, remembers the days of the Sanatorium Board's big white trucks very clearly from his youth in the late 1950s, shortly after the start of Jim Zayshley's career:

> I remember it was an occasion. I remember seeing that long white truck pull into town in the afternoon. It didn't scare me, but there was something sickly and ominous about its whiteness. One grew a little more alert. I knew TB was serious stuff.
>
> They parked on the lot of the old high school in Steinbach, not to x-ray only students, but as many people in town as they could. I remember lineups at one end of the trailer, people going in to get their x-ray, then leaving by a back exit. It was set up so you walked through a kind of assembly line inside the trailer. This happened once a year. My memory tells me it was a long trailer, and a cab at the front. All white. I do remember that the last few times this truck arrived, it wasn't for x-rays but to give us TB shots [skin tests] to show the presence of TB.
>
> This happened for three or four years, then the trucks just vanished. I guess TB disappeared at that time. I remember the humming sound of the truck. A generator, I imagine. Inside, the x-rays made a sound too, at least that's how it seems to me now.

Steinbach, a town of about 2,500 at that time, was not unique in receiving these high-profile visits from the San Board's big white trucks. They went everywhere. In Winnipeg, local celebrities like Blue Bombers quarterback Don Jonas had his chest x-ray done to publicize the importance of being checked for TB as late as 1974.

One of the things Jim Zayshley did through the 1950s and '60s was show educational films about TB in community halls and churches all over Manitoba. It was part of spreading the word. One of the films he showed most was *The Road to Recovery*. The film spells out the goal of the Manitoba Sanatorium at Ninette, and also the Board's goal, the "control and ultimate eradication of TB." Drug therapy is discussed, but the san and the surgeon are clearly preferred options. The mobile units, in all their clean white glory, are prominent, referred to as "traveling chest clinics." Jim Zayshley himself makes a cameo appearance as a young x-ray technician.

There can be no doubt from watching this film that the people who made it considered the content to be critical information for everyone in their society. Like the trucks, this film was for the mass-market. The predominantly white middle class was still very aware of tuberculosis – they saw it as a disease that anyone could get, including them. They did not see TB as something that only affected people who were different from them, socially marginalized.

ROMANCING THE COUGH

Back when TB was on the minds of the middle class, we told ourselves stories about glamorous artists and characters who got the disease. What these stories about famous TB victims really demonstrate is simply that many people died of TB in the industrialized world, especially in the 19th and early 20th centuries. In the 19th century, the normal way of looking at TB was what René Dubos called an "attitude of perverted sentimentalism." Perhaps this was a natural reaction to something so appalling and out of control that people coped psychologically by romanticizing the disease.

TB was at epidemic proportions in Europe throughout the 18th and 19th centuries, and the epidemic spread to the new world colonies. In the early 18th century, TB caused about one-third of all the deaths in Europe, making it the number one killer. The cure rate for TB patients in Victorian England was under 3%. In the 19th century, as Mother Europe exported industrial civilization and disease to America, one fifth of all the deaths in the United States were caused by TB, and the number in Europe was still one-seventh. In Canada, TB was one of the ten leading causes of death through the Second World War. Overwhelmingly, the disease struck the young: children, young adults, and pregnant women. About half of those who got active cases of TB died within five years. This was true well into the 20th century and the great era of the TB sanatorium. In an awful irony, Edward Livingstone Trudeau died of tuberculosis in 1915, the doctor whose pioneering TB sanatorium in upstate New York inspired the building of the Ninette San and countless others. Little wonder that fantasy coloured people's perception of the disease – reality was just too grim, and illness had to be transformed into romantic metaphor.

Glamorization of the disease came long before the first effective control of TB through public health measures and later the advent of antibiotic treatment. For the Victorians especially, who associated disease with artistic sensitivity, the list of tuberculous brilliance is long. Among the 19th century writers who died of the disease are John Keats, Emily and Charlotte Brontë, Robert Louis Stevenson, and Anton Chekhov. These authors were glamour victims of the disease, pale, wasted and often young.

Alexandre Dumas *fils* fixed the image of tuberculosis in the public mind as a disease of the sensitive, physically fragile and sexually passionate. The protagonist of his novel and play *Camille (La Dame aux Camilias)* is Marguerite Gautier, who later became Verdi's Violetta in the opera *La Traviata*, and she is the romantic embodiment of a consumptive – a TB patient. She is rail-thin, languidly feverish, and highly sympathetic even though she's a prostitute. In the narrative she suffers from the "disease of love," a euphemism for TB. She is euphoric with both sexual longing and the awareness that she must soon die: it was a common belief that TB increased the capacity for euphoria and creative achievement even as it shortened the consumptive's life. Only by withdrawing entirely from the excitement of one's over-sensitized life could anyone hope to survive the disease. This was perfect cultural conditioning for public acceptance of rest therapy and sanatoria, even if Dumas and Verdi never intended that. In 1936, at the height of the sanatorium era, the image of the anorexic Marguerite was captured for a new generation when Greta Garbo played her in the movie version of *Camille*.

The English romantic poet John Keats was a real-life celebrity victim of tuberculosis. He famously wrote, in his poem "Ode to a Nightingale," about the time "where youth grows pale, and spectre-thin, and dies." What many don't know is that Keats trained for six years as a doctor, and diagnosed himself when he first coughed up blood about a year before his death: "That is arterial blood, I cannot be deceived in that colour. It is my death warrant." Keats died in 1821 at the age of 26, a victim of what was then called galloping consumption: his disease did not canter or hesitate, it galloped to its fatal conclusion. Keats likely got the disease from either his mother or his brother, each of whom he spent a year nursing before they died of TB. He slept in the same room as his brother Tom for months on end. Like many TB victims to this day, close confinement with a relative led directly to his demise.

Robert Louis Stevenson, the author of *Jekyll and Hyde* and *Treasure Island*, died of TB in Samoa in 1894. Unlike Keats, he lived with the disease for many years before he succumbed. If he'd lived in the age of the airplane he would have left behind a lifetime's worth of air miles with his globe-trotting attempts to find a climate that would allow him to breathe. Even in the late 19th century, after Robert Koch had demonstrated that TB was caused by a germ, doctors were still recommending that patients live in warm climates or mountainous ones or take sea voyages in the hope that this would somehow cleanse their lungs. Stevenson was impatient with the medical profession, which may well have helped him survive for more than three decades with an active case of TB.

The Russian writer Anton Chekhov chose to ignore medical advice about his TB near the turn of the 20th century even though he himself was trained as a doctor. In 1897 Chekhov wrote to his brother, "Since 1884 I have been spitting blood every spring." Yet he never consulted a physician until his collapse that same year, and unlike Stevenson, Chekhov did not attempt treatment by travel to warmer climes. Instead he smoked, wrote volumes of short stories and plays, and occasionally practised medicine. He died in 1904 at age 44.

By the 20th century the arts were no longer helping to romance the cough of TB. For example, the Italian artist Amadeo Modigliani painted about 200 portraits between 1916 and 1919 many of which feature oval-shaped faces that reflect the ravages of TB, the wasting disease. Modigliani, a serious alcoholic, suffered horribly with TB and died of it in 1920, aged 36. His pregnant wife reacted by throwing herself out of a window to her death. No one could romanticize the death of Franz Kafka either. He had TB of the larynx by the 1920s, and the only medical care was palliative. It consisted of painful twice-daily injections of alcohol directly into Kafka's larynx.

In 1952, René and Jean Dubos wrote in their classic text *The White Plague: Tuberculosis, Man, and Society,* that "little by little, it dawned on social common sense what a mockery it was to depict consumption as a spiritualization of the being, as a romantic experience detached from the horrid aspects of disease." It is perhaps no coincidence that René Dubos, world-famous as an antibiotic researcher by 1940, was able to write about "social common sense" and TB in the year 1952. René's first wife Marie Louise had died of TB, and Jean, his second wife and frequent collaborator, would only survive her infection thanks to the antibiotic revolution that her husband's work helped make possible. Thanks to effective drug therapy, millions of lives would be saved from the white plague of TB in the second half of the 20th century. Calm rationality in the face of a curable disease is vastly easier to maintain than when there is no cure, as the recent hysteria blaming autism on childhood vaccination demonstrates.

Oscar Wilde wrote that "one must have a heart of stone to read the death of [the Charles Dickens character] Little Nell without laughing," and it's easy to feel the same way about Greta Garbo's romantic version of TB in the movie *Camille.* However, it is not just that we have become too sophisticated for *Camille.* More than anything else modern public health measures and medical science have made the romantic story of TB seem foolish to us. But our smug laughter is premature, and TB has not gone away.

BACK ON MAIN STREET

So while the glamour victims of tuberculosis still took centre stage until well into the 20th century, the real victims lived and died in much less romantic conditions, not only in urban Europe but in the colonized new world too. That included Winnipeg, Gateway to the West, the city that saw itself as destined to be an intercontinental railway hub until the Panama Canal shattered that dream by providing cheaper transportation to the Pacific in 1913.

The people who died of TB were the same impoverished, overcrowded people who die of TB today, in the developing world — and in Winnipeg. But in the 19th century, diseases that we now associate with the developing world were right here in Canada, because we were the developing world. From about 1880 until the First World War, Winnipeg hosted outbreaks of typhoid fever, smallpox, tuberculosis, venereal disease, scarlet fever, and diphtheria. These outbreaks and epidemics, though, were often invisible to those with money and status. Those who suffered most from overcrowded housing and poor sanitation were immigrants living in the North End of the city. Almost half the houses in the North End were not connected to the city waterworks system. According to a 1904 doctor's report to city council, Winnipeg had over 6,500 "box closets" for toilets, even on Main Street and Portage Avenue. "Box closets" were outdoor toilets made of a wooden box set on top of the ground and they were not necessarily watertight. The same report said that "the filth, squalor, and overcrowding among the foreign elements is beyond our power of description." The doctor's report goes on to make this simple but rather prophetic statement:

> It must be remembered, however, that in sanitary matters the welfare of one section of the city is inseparably connected with that of another. The interests of the community so far as public health is concerned are not restricted by geographical or social boundaries.

In 1900 there had already been a serious outbreak of smallpox, and then the city reacted by sending patients to a "pest house" near the edge of town. The pest house was conveniently located 100 yards from a cemetery. Patients who wanted to escape were shackled, and clergymen read the last rites upwind of the grave. By 1906 Winnipeg had its worst-ever typhoid outbreak and was the typhoid capital of North America; this is a disease nearly always caused by water supplies polluted with sewage.

By 1913 the North End of Winnipeg had a 25% infant mortality rate, while the south and west ends, populated by the merchant and middle classes, had about half that. Sadly for those North End residents, it seems that only the city's health department saw a connection between these statistics and the provision of adequate housing and sewage. Politicians were unwilling to take action, choosing instead to blame the victims. Winnipeg's Anglo-Saxon establishment saw the immigrants who populated the North End as simply lazy and ignorant, "not of a desirable class," as the *Dominion* newspaper put it in 1912.

In 1911 the city's new health officer, Dr. A.J. Douglas, wrote that he knew of "no question of more vital importance to the future welfare of the city than the housing problem."[1] The Winnipeg health department was more concerned about urban decay than were the civic politicians or prominent citizens. How had this come about?

---

[1] In one of history's many strange ironies, Dr. Douglas, one of the most important doctors responsible for improving Winnipeg's public health, was the son of the original owner of the Leland Hotel. While it was a luxury hotel in 1900, by the end of the twentieth century it had become a skid row joint behind its elegant façade, and it was frequently visited by the Manitoba Lung Association's TB survey team. It burned down in January 1999.

THERE GOES THE NEIGHBOURHOOD

Anyone who visits Winnipeg today and drives over the Red River on the Disraeli Freeway will wonder why the surrounding area looks like a festering industrial slum. The answer is simple. Starting in 1895, Point Douglas, protruding into a hairpin curve of the Red River like the snout of a bearskin on broad-shouldered Winnipeg, was bisected right down the middle by the scar of the CPR main line railway. The train tracks divided the city into North and South, immigrants and Anglo-Saxons, workers and managers, have-nots and haves. The railway brought jobs and profits to the merchants who supplied settlers in the expanding west from their Exchange-area warehouses. But because of the lack of public transit across the main line to the north for many years, the railroad also made the social and health problems of the "foreigners" in the North End largely invisible to those who lived in the rest of Winnipeg. It's hard to take seriously problems that you never see.

By the turn of the century, Winnipeg's core area had single-family homes being turned into squalid rooming houses. Point Douglas became an industrial neighbourhood with the coming of the railway, and so all the luxurious brick houses of the city's early elite were converted into businesses, rooming houses and sometimes brothels. There was now rot at the city's centre, largely invisible to the middle and upper classes who controlled civic politics.

Alan Artibise, an urban studies professor and historian, has told the story of how the railway's placement ended up marring Winnipeg's economic and social development. Winnipeg city council, in a desperate bid to make sure that Sir John A. Macdonald's federal government did not route the CPR line through Selkirk, offered inducements that went beyond what was necessary to ensure the main trunk went through Winnipeg. As Artibise puts it, the city politicians

> gave the companies [railways] a free hand to enter and leave Winnipeg at their convenience. They thus left to future generations of Winnipeggers a poor legacy, for geography, railroads, and a blind commitment to growth combined to turn Winnipeg's environment into an uncoordinated and socially disruptive series of self-contained ghettos.

Corporate welfare is as much part of Winnipeg history as the Red River. The city, starting in the 1880s, invested heavily in attracting railways, and also built a city-owned hydro plant. In addition it campaigned actively to attract the same immigrants who suffered from inadequate housing and health care once they arrived. What Artibise calls "the growth ethic of Winnipeg's commercial elite" meant that almost no one considered the city planning or public health issues associated with uncontrolled growth.

One of the primary ways that the business class ensured its political domination was by maintaining property qualifications for municipal voters. Candidates needed to own at least $2,000 in property, and voters somewhat less.

These rules disenfranchised the majority of Winnipeg citizens. For example, in 1906, there were 7,784 registered municipal voters in a population of about 100,000. The other significant political development for the working poor in Winnipeg was the re-drawing of city wards in 1920, right on the heels of the Winnipeg General Strike. Ward 5, which included Point Douglas and most of central Winnipeg, had always voted for labour candidates. Collapsing seven wards, including Ward 5, into three diluted the labour vote and effectively removed political representation from this area.

When elites make policy decisions the outcomes are not equitable, but they're also not accidental. Alan Artibise spoke to me about how resource allocation in city planning is deliberate:

> Whatever city you go to, if you drive around different neighbourhoods and look at public service – whether the streets are clean, whether the garbage is picked up, what kind of parks they have – it's not random. Theoretically services should be the same throughout the city, but they never are. I would argue that these are conscious decisions about how resources are allocated. It's no accident that school participation rates, crime, and disease, are not randomly distributed either but are related to how policies are conceived and implemented. As I drive around New Orleans, where I live now, there are areas in the city where they don't pick up the garbage. Segregation is not an accidental policy, whether it's segregation of services, or of race, ethnicity or economic status.

In 1909 civic officials in Winnipeg decided to segregate prostitution and the social and health problems that go with it in the Point Douglas area. The area was chosen deliberately by city officials as a vice district, since the affluent and politically influential were now living elsewhere. The Point Douglas brothels at their peak numbered about 53 and were concentrated on McFarlane and Rachel (now called Annabella). The area was suitable because while its residents were respectable and hard-working, many of them were also disenfranchised immigrants who would never complain. There were no zoning hearings to approve this unofficial decision. The brothel operators were also satisfied with the arrangement, since their establishments were in walking distance of the CPR station and the booming Main Street hotel strip. As for well-to-do Winnipeg, out of sight meant out of mind. According to Alan Artibise, the brothels kept operating for "a full thirty years until the trade fell victim to amateur competition during the depression." Prostitutes frequent the area to this day.

WE'RE ALL CONNECTED

In early winter I drive into Point Douglas and park near the Disraeli Freeway. The Disraeli rips through Point Douglas like a giant zipper, or maybe more like the railway that originally divided Winnipeg into two distinct societies. I'm here to visit Sage House, a program that provides medical and social services to female sex trade workers, transgender individuals, and their children.

Sage House is located in a decaying two-and-a-half-story house just off the Disraeli Freeway. I get escorted quickly through the house because men aren't really supposed to visit here. There is a sparsely furnished but cozy living room with a TV set, a big clean kitchen, and a rack of medical pamphlets. A surprising number of these are about TB. The floors of the house twist up and down as if they were surfing a flood plain, and they are. Sage House will have to move to a building that's in better shape soon, somewhere in the same area.

Sage House operates a drop-in program on weekday afternoons and two evenings a week there are prepared meals for clients. There are laundry facilities and outreach workers who offer counseling services and provide links to other social services. Sage House works from what they describe as a philosophy of "non-judgmental harm reduction" for the people they work with. The organization was originally called POWER (Prostitutes and Other Women for Equal Rights). Then it was part of Street Connection, which still runs a van offering condoms, a needle exchange, and the *Street News* newspaper to the same clientele. The needle exchange program is now run out of Nine Circles at the former site of one of Winnipeg's two great railway hotels. Sage House is operated by Mount Carmel Clinic, which has provided health care to disadvantaged people in Winnipeg's North End since 1926.

June Friesen[2] started working at Sage House in 1996. She was a nurse in Repulse Bay before then for about five years. Sage House wanted someone who had worked up north, since many of their clients are from northern communities. June dealt with lots of people who'd been in TB sanatoria, and Earl Hershfield had seen many of them. "Lots of the Inuit over 50 have been in a san."

"Many of our clients are street-involved," says June, and a few of them are trying to get out of their street involvement. The clients have substance abuse problems and a lot are either homeless or have low-quality housing. Many of the clients are Aboriginal, and some of them are transgender, living as if their sex was different from their biology. "It's a population that's not accessing much medical care outside of emergency rooms," says June, but "they're actually a very resilient bunch of people."

June offers clients whatever nursing services they need: she does pregnancy testing, PAP smears, urine testing for bladder infections, and provides birth control and advice. "There are lots of other health issues that come up which are blended with social issues," she says. Sometimes she wishes people would go to doctors or hospitals, but many clients don't even have health cards.

TB case-finding and treatments happen regularly at Sage House. The Manitoba Lung Association's x-ray survey team comes here on a regular basis.

---

[2] Not her real name.

Their last visit was just a few months earlier, when they x-rayed 15 or 20 people, including staff. The survey team offered a draw for $50 cash as an incentive to clients to get x-rayed, and that worked well. There is of course a concern about co-infection with TB and HIV. "It almost always seems like somebody's cousin is in the hospital with TB," says June. Not only has she dealt with the more common pulmonary (infectious) TB, but in 1996 June administered a year's supply of drug therapy for a client with meningeal TB. Later she had another patient who had a less formal version of directly observed therapy: a bartender at a Main Street Hotel gave meds to a patient with her beer.

I ask June what she thinks the public should know about her clients.

I think people should know that economics forces people into crowded living situations and not caring for their health because of whatever else takes over. It forces people into situations that they become accustomed to, and you think 'why is somebody choosing this,' but they're not really choosing it at all. I feel silly sometimes trying to deal with the medical issues when the root of them is social.

Then I ask her why people in the larger community should be concerned about the health of her clients. She says: "We are all connected, and the connections are endless. It would be foolish to think that we shouldn't care about problems that we only see some of us having."

6

ANOTHER COUNTRY

Visiting a First Nation in northern Manitoba is like going to a foreign country for someone like me, a white member of the Canadian middle class who lives in the city and knows about the north only second-hand. Language, culture, landscape, even the weather is different. It starts with the airline. I call them weeks in advance to reserve a flight. Turns out you can reserve your flight but cancel anytime before the plane leaves – nothing goes on your credit card until you get a boarding pass. This flexibility is good because I need permission both from the First Nation and the federal government to visit the community's nursing station, and it isn't really clear to me who makes a final decision or when. You can change your schedule at a moment's notice if something – most likely the weather – changes. No one asks for ID or checks your baggage for box-cutters.

On a chilly late winter morning I board the plane. The airline operates a fleet of twin-propped Fairchild Metro 11 aircraft affectionately known by northern travelers as "flying pencils," since that's how they look. The 18-seat cabin is pressurized and the planes cruise at about 300 miles an hour. On this flight the co-pilot also acts as stewardess, and her main job before take-off is to shout out the schedule over the engine noise, and then hand out yellow plastic earplugs for the journey. Turns out the engines get a lot louder once you're in the air. We climb sharply over Winnipeg's sprawling river-twisted grid and turn north.

Once we're at cruising altitude it's like we're high above a beach of white clouds, although the noise is continuous and jarring, even with the yellow plugs jammed in your ears. The vague outlines of lake, ice and forest are faintly visible sometimes, and everybody settles back to read newspapers. The *Winnipeg Free Press* has a story about a new report that says Aboriginal and poor people are the least healthy in Canada, with statistics that approach "third world" conditions. First Nations people on-reserve have a 21% chance of getting tuberculosis, compared to 1.3% for the rest of Canadians. Obesity, smoking, and diabetes are all at very high rates on-reserve as well.

When I look up from the newspaper the boreal forest below us is more visible. We are close to our destination. The descent takes us through wisps of cloud that are like the ones I've seen at the Health Sciences Centre on the chest x-rays of patients with tuberculosis in their lungs. But no one could really think of this landscape as diseased; looking out the window I see an island that looks like a black forest chocolate cake oozing rich white cream where splotches of exposed earth are surrounded by snow and ice. A sunburst splits one of the props in the stiff morning air. Then suddenly we are in the forest among tree tips and landing on a lake and it's as if a curtain ripped aside to reveal a perfect diorama of spruce and pine. I can see houses and trucks and a microwave tower nestled around the edges of the lake.

I get out of the plane and walk out into blinding sunshine that rolls off the snow and ice. The airport is a small single story building with one big room and a couple of smaller ones. The walls are cheap, scuffed paneling decorated with a couple of bulletin boards and a poster advertising Health Canada's Aboriginal Diabetes Initiative. Everyone has told me to be patient here, but I immediately start pacing in a tight circle with my backpack – someone was supposed to pick me up and show me around. In about five minutes he shows up: a tall, parka-heavy man approaches and says, you're here about Dr. Hershfield? I say yes and follow him outside. He's from the nursing station and is not the guide I expected, but he will give me a ride to the motel so I can check in.

My ride is a yellow plastic sled pulled behind an ATV. I get in with a Health Canada psychologist named Roy[3] who was on the flight from Winnipeg. Roy has taken this ride before and sits gingerly on the edge of the sled. I sit what looks like a bench in the sled. The ride is bone-jarring even at low speed around corners and across the lake to the nursing station and community-owned motel. The driver lets me out at the motel and points out the band office, a low white shed that should be within walking distance across another part of the lake.

There is no one visible from the desk when I enter the motel. It's clean and pleasant, and there are two felt-marker signs posted: one says "No intoxicated people allowed in these premises" and the other says "Cigarettes go up $1.50 per package at 9 pm. ABSOLUTELY no credit." There is a lounge to the right with a TV set and a number of ashtrays under no smoking signs, and a restaurant. I walk into the restaurant and find someone sweeping up. She nods at me and walks to the front desk in measured steps, handing me a form to fill in. Do you need a credit card imprint? I ask. Oh no.

The motel room is perfectly clean and comfortable but comes with an odd set of absences. There is no garbage can or Kleenex. There are no drawer pulls on the chest of drawers, just sharp screws jutting out. There is no Gideon Bible. I drop my

---

[3] Names of people in the community have been changed throughout this chapter.

back-pack on the bed, dump out the extra clothes, and leave the motel for a hike to the band office. The chief promised me a guide and since there's no evidence of one, I'll go see the chief.

The view walking down to the lake from the motel and the nursing station is breathtaking. It's like a Tom Thompson painting that was never done, maybe never quite imagined, with huge pine trees stark against the lightly rolling water, then the ice, and a few decaying swings hanging from spruce trees in the foreground. Across from the motel is a one-floor apartment building that houses the community's elders. I walk past the elder house on a snowmobile track and start sinking in the snow as I approach the lake. Then there's noise behind me, someone on a snowmobile. A serious looking man with a thick moustache says, Where you going? To the band office. Same here, you want a ride? I jump behind him and we glide across the lake.

WAITING

The band office looks like a run-down garage on the outside, with faded metal doors and an old hand-lettered sign in Cree. Inside it's paneled with fake wood-grain. When you walk into the office there is a large spread of cardboard where people take off their boots and shoes. The first thing you see when your boots come off is a framed photo of the original signatories to the treaty the band falls under, signed in 1909 by three very grim-looking men who stare directly into the camera. There are photocopies of other old pictures taped on the walls. Some of them are half torn-down, and one has been defaced with the addition of facial hair on women and children in the picture, so they match the man's facial hair.

The guy who gave me a ride asks who I want to see. Chief Beardy, I say. Oh, he's in a meeting. Just walk in. That's what everyone does. This feels very wrong to me. I'm already an outsider, a "reporter" as Chief Beardy calls me, "media" as the government people say. I won't be walking into any meetings.

So I cool my heels and look around. On the bulletin board in the front is a June 2003 "public notice" that says that acts of vandalism by members of the community will result in deductions from welfare or payroll, and criminal charges. If the vandals can't pay, they will have to work off the damage they do. Parents will be held responsible for their children's actions. "The above action is taken with honorable intent to keep our community safe and free from fear of willful damage." There's also a sign that warns people not to barge into the chief and council office. It says "Please don't come into the chief and council office if no one is present because of confidential issues on the desks." Obviously Chief Beardy's constituents don't have the same scruples I do, but of course they're not white media guys from the south.

There's a northern newspaper sitting on the table beside me called *The Drum*. A headline announces that winter roads are ready – with an early spring coming this is a mighty short season for road access. Of the two dozen First Nation communities north of Lake Winnipeg, about half have access only by air and winter roads. Building materials, among other things, can only come into these communities by road. One other story catches my eye, this one headlined "Manitoba First Nations Debt Nearly One-third National Total." The reason for this disproportionate share of debt in Manitoba, acknowledged by the federal government, is that First Nations here are incurring debt to build new houses and schools.

There's a stir in the hallway and someone comes out carrying an overhead projector. I take a guess at which of the men in the hall is Chief Beardy. My second guess is correct. He says that one of the community health workers will show me around, and that he can see me later in the afternoon. I introduce myself to the man with the projector, who turns out to be a community nurse, and he drives me back to the motel.

NURSING STATION

Virtually all the lunches at the motel involve hamburgers, hot dogs and French fries (which cost extra). The radio is an Aboriginal station that broadcasts in Cree and plays a lot of Shania Twain. I start out sitting by myself in one of the booths made out of laminate on metal frames but then Roy the psychologist waves me over. Roy is interested in the fact that I'm a writer. He is writing a book himself – a self-help book for people with psychological problems. Roy wants my advice for how he can finish his book, find an agent, and make a lot of money. He can't tell me much about the book because his theory about human nature is so new and unique that he needs to guard it closely.

After lunch I walk across the road to the nursing station. The community health nurse, Jonathan, is new. He shows me the room where he sees patients. There are two large posters from the CDC in Atlanta on the walls that say "Think TB" in large letters and then list all the major symptoms of tuberculosis. There is also a sign that lists in large type the side effects of one of the major TB drugs: vomiting, yellow urine, headache, joint pain, etc. There is a community TB registry on Jonathan's desk, and a thick file labeled "TB skin tests to be read." On a shelf is a "Clinician's Guide" to TB. Other than in books and Earl Hershfield's offices in Winnipeg, I have never seen so many signs that TB is not a history exhibit.

The actual interview with Jonathan and the other nurses cannot begin until the head nurse, Joyce, is available. After about half an hour Joyce and another nurse take us into a lounge with a satellite TV, a table, and a large couch. Joyce shuts off the TV, closes all the doors, and puts a document on the table. I have already talked to the Media Relations people at the First Nations and Inuit Health Branch (FNIHB) office in Winnipeg, who operate this nursing station on behalf of the federal government. They will only allow me to ask questions in advance, in writing, and the nurses will only respond in writing. So we spend a rather stilted hour going over their written responses to my questions. I'm not allowed to run a recorder.

TB is a mandatory community health program under the area of communicable disease control provided by FNIHB. The local health team, which consists of a couple of nurses, a few community health representatives, and a visiting doctor, are responsible for reporting cases of TB and helping with contact tracing. Contact tracing means finding out whom TB-infected patients have been in contact with, since the disease is spread by infectious people as they cough and breathe.

Owen is the "direct observation therapist," which in TB control jargon means someone whose job is making sure that people take their pills, which you do by "directly observing" them swallow their medication. This is a very important job. One of the big problems with treating TB is that patients need to take a cocktail of unpleasant drugs over an extended period of time – currently about 9 months. So Owen schedules patient visits, coordinates rides for them since the community is scattered, and actually observes them taking their meds ("direct observation"). Owen was originally a security guard at the nursing station. He noticed that TB patients came in after hours through a separate entrance to get their medication, and he often volunteered to help out with these patients. After a couple of years budget was available and he was hired to be a direct observation therapist instead of a guard.

The provincial TB control program itself is operated by a division of the Manitoba Lung Association, and FNIHB contracts with the provincial Lung Association to provide TB control services in First Nations communities. Until recently, the Medical Director of the TB control program was Dr. Earl Hershfield. For 37 years he personally read every x-ray and made recommendations on treatment for anyone diagnosed with TB in Manitoba. The people at this nursing station have only spoken to him on the phone. Owen asked me to bring a picture of Dr. Hershfield, because he was curious what he looked like. The TB control presence in communities like this one came from Joann MacMorran, who was the Nurse Consultant for TB Control in Dr. Hershfield's program since 1971. Joann visited this First Nation and others many times. Joyce has met her and so has Owen. In addition to the program run by the Manitoba Lung Association, FNIHB also has its own TB nurse and a program to control TB in First Nations communities. Like many parts of our health care system, responsibility and jurisdiction are complicated, especially with regards to First Nations. For the last four decades there's no doubt that the TB control program has been highly effective in Manitoba. The number of active cases among Aboriginal people in the province now is about half what it was in the 1970s. In communities like this one, though, the numbers don't tell the whole story.

The political leadership in First Nations is gradually taking over responsibility for health care, education, and all community programs. For now, Chief and Council in the community appoint a Health Councillor, and the band council works with FNIHB and the TB control program to ensure the right decisions are made and everyone's in the loop. At least that's the theory. As I find out later, reality is not exactly the same as what would go on a Power Point presentation in Winnipeg that keeps using the words "consult" and "collaborate."

TUBERCULOSIS SCREENING AND TREATMENT

The four of us, Joyce, the head nurse, Jonathan, Owen and I sit around a battered kitchen table and Joyce keeps reading from their document. I asked them how much time they spend contact tracing for TB, and the answer is so much they don't even count the hours. This community happens to have the highest rate of TB in the province, and has for about 20 years. So a lot of time at the nursing station goes into tracing the contacts of anyone who tests positive for TB. In a small community like this – the on-reserve population is about 1,300 – if there are 11 active cases, they might each have 25 contacts, so that means 275 people will be screened for TB, a significant chunk of the population.

Screening begins with patients at the clinic who have TB symptoms – Joyce always calls them "clients." If a client has symptoms – a persistent cough or cold, weight loss, pneumonia-like symptoms – one of the nurses takes a chest x-ray and it goes to Winnipeg for reading by a physician in the TB unit. A skin test is taken and read after 48 hours and 72 hours; this involves injecting a protein substance that contains a tiny amount of TB germ to see if there's a reaction. Any swelling of the skin area larger than ten millimetres where the injection was made means that the patient may be infected with TB. Skin tests and result interpretations get faxed to the TB unit. Sputum (spit) samples are collected and sent out to Cadham Lab in Winnipeg and results come back within a week. Cultures can take up to two weeks for a report. So positive screening can be a positive skin test, an abnormal chest x-ray, or a sputum sample that comes back positive for TB germs or bacilli. If screening is positive then a doctor in the TB unit decides on a treatment plan, and it might take from two weeks to a month before they issue that plan.

Based on the doctor's recommendation, a client who has screened positive for TB is sent south to Winnipeg to the Health Sciences Centre Respiratory Hospital. For many Aboriginal people this is the first time they have gone south or been in a city. At the hospital, drug treatment begins immediately. The nursing staff initiates contact tracing right away too. Clients are usually in the hospital for two to three weeks and are not released until repeated sputum samples test as negative for TB. Then they fly back to their community to continue treatment under the nursing station's supervision.

Tuberculosis is unusual among infectious diseases because you can be infected without having active disease. Medical people call this LTBI, or "latent TB infection." When a skin test for TB shows that someone has LTBI, they are often given preventive treatment with a plan that comes from the central office in Winnipeg. The nursing station goes over the plan with the patient.

At the nursing station, they interview the client and go over the treatment plan to get their agreement. Then they do a liver function test for a pre-treatment baseline, since TB drugs are hard on the liver. There's a budget for juice, crackers, jam and so on for people taking TB medicine, since the drugs are hard to take. Clients come in to take their medication under observation at the nursing station twice a week. Every time they come in and take medicine Owen records the date and time and signs off. The nursing station runs an appointment system for the TB program, and the band provides transportation for people to come in to take their medicine.

THE LOCAL TB PROGRAM

"IT WAS ONLY ONCE THE NURSING STATIONS GOT INVOLVED THAT THERE WAS SOME
RAPPORT WITH THE PEOPLE ON RESERVES AND THEN WE STARTED TO SUCCEED."
— EARL HERSHFIELD

It is clear that Joyce is proud of their work on TB. They are doing an annual TB screening program in the community that last year did chest x-rays on 837 people. The school screening program does skin testing in grades one and six. When clients miss appointments and don't take their medicine, the nursing station works with them to solve whatever the problem is: sometimes they need a babysitter, sometimes the problem is side effects from the drugs. They have never had to invoke the Public Health Act and force compliance with a band constable or the RCMP, but that would be the last resort.

The nursing station does an enormous amount of record keeping for TB control. They issue a monthly report to the TB control program in Winnipeg. They record medication dosages, side effects, whether medicine is crushed, mixed with jam, and so on. Missed doses and appointments have to be recorded. There is a community TB registry, both on paper and on computer, and it lists all test results. There is a "hot list" of contacts for follow-up. Community statistics are kept and presented to Chief and Council.

Educational activities are one of the things they are doing more now. Jonathan invites me to a presentation he's giving at an elementary school tomorrow. He and Owen just gave a presentation to Chief and Council this morning, and they plan to talk to the police, the Northern Store, and Hydro. Community radio stations are also broadcasting information pieces about TB in Cree and English.

If someone with TB leaves or returns to the community, then the nursing station immediately informs Winnipeg's TB control program, who maintain a registry of cases. If the person's location is unknown, the nursing station staff will make inquiries among family members and friends. The idea is to prevent any delay in treatment or contact tracing.

WHY HERE?

I asked Joyce how living up north is different from life in the south. She wrote that "it's like comparing apples and oranges – there is no comparison between southern and northern communities. They are totally different." I also asked her why there are so often outbreaks of TB in northern communities. At this point she starts to say more than what's in the document, becoming quite animated. She talks about the isolation, the lack of jobs and recreational activity, poor housing, nutrition, and sanitation, and the high cost of living. Joyce observes that air freight costs 89 cents a pound and that return air fare to Winnipeg is about $500. Groceries, clothing, hydro and fuel all cost much more than they do in the south.

I also asked Joyce about why there are repeated outbreaks of TB in her community. She talks about housing. Poor ventilation systems in houses mean that TB is "easily spread." There is overcrowding, with two or three families living in a single house. Lung disease is exacerbated because of people using wood stoves when they can't afford electric or fuel heating.

The cost of sewage and running water is high, says Joyce. The community is built on clay and bedrock, and so it's difficult to install plumbing and sewage. At this point Paul, a community health rep, speaks up. He says "honey buckets" or "slob pails," five gallon plastic pails, are still used for toilets in many households. He seems both amused and grim about this.

Joyce talks about the difficulty of recruiting and retaining professional staff in a remote community. A doctor visits only two days a week. Community health nurses have to be on-call continuously and there's a high rate of burn-out. A dentist comes 10 days a month and there is an annual eye clinic.

Because there isn't enough recreational activity this causes other problems, says Joyce, like a "high rate of suicide attempts, alcohol and substance abuse, and gambling problems." There are three churches (Catholic, United, and Pentecostal) in the community, competing for people's souls while ignoring their bodies. I've seen a letter in the United Church archive in Winnipeg about this community, noting in 1968 that there is "little or no recreation for young people on the reserve." Part of the reason there was so little recreation was that Sunday nights were considered too holy by most of the church leaders for anything other than worship, and Sunday nights were also the safest night of the week for people to come out, since there was less drinking in the community on the seventh day.

WHAT THEY DIDN'T KNOW

I get a ride back to the band office with Paul in his truck. He talks about how hard the roads are on truck suspensions. I ask him if he thinks winter is almost over, and he laughs and refuses to speculate. I sit down again at the front of the band office and wait for Chief Beardy. After almost two hours, the Chief and one of his councillors invite me in to the band's meeting room to sit at a long table with orange plastic chairs. There is a stuffed pickerel on the wall and a number of large survey maps behind me, and I sit facing windows that look out on the pristine lake and the winter road. There is really only one thing they want to tell me today, so my interview script is irrelevant.

The Chief says that he and Council were shocked to learn that their community had more new cases of infectious tuberculosis than anywhere else in the province, and also had the second-highest TB incidence in Canada. They found out only about a year ago, when someone from Health Canada gave the Band Council a presentation and told them about their incidence rate. In 2003, they had 15 active cases in a population of 1,300. The Canadian average rate for 2003 was 5.5 per 100,000 people. If this community were average for TB incidence and had 15 cases, there would be about 250,000 people living here.

"Why did they withhold this information from us?" says Chief Beardy. "What kind of people would do that?"

My first reaction, internally, is skepticism. How could they not have known this? It's a matter of public record. My second reaction is defensive, because now they are asking me why I wanted to visit their community.

"Did you come because you heard about the TB here?"

"Well, yes. Part of the story is the high amount of TB in the north."

"And so how did you know about the TB in our community?"

"Well, Dr. Hershfield mentioned it to me, and I just went to the university library and looked it up."

What I mean to say is that the information is in the public domain. You can search for "tuberculosis and Manitoba" in a university library and come up with research that tracks TB incidence by community. But I was forgetting something.

"We have no library here," says Chief Beardy. I look at him, and his face is framed by the vast emptiness of the lake and the darkening horizon behind him. He seems angry. Is he playing some kind of political game, I wonder. He has only been Chief for four years though. I remember how reluctant he was to talk to me in the first place, when I called over and over again from Winnipeg. He's right. There is no library here. And if the previous Chief knew, well, if there's no institutional memory in Ottawa, why should there be any here in a tiny place struggling for survival?

MOTEL

I get a ride back to the motel and head to my room. In the hallway is a Natural Resources Canada map of Manitoba. Natural Resources issues maps that show First Nation lands, or reserves, together with national parks. It's as if they think the reserves and the parks are both tourist attractions. There was a time when Indian Health Services, the precursor to the First Nations and Inuit Health Branch, was part of the Department of Mines and Resources. So back then First Nations were considered either mines or resources.

The only phone available is a pay telephone in the lobby, and I use that to call home after dinner. The television set in the room only gets CBC, and the evening news features a story on Aboriginal hip-hop artists, the 2004 version of Aboriginal cowboy singers. Having one channel is boring so I go out to the lobby where they have a satellite-equipped TV set. Roy and the security guard are watching "To Serve and Protect," a Canadian show that features hapless Canucks running afoul of the law, often with much bleeping on the soundtrack. The motel security guard tells me that recently the show featured someone from the community getting arrested on-camera. Tonight we see an intoxicated Vancouver prostitute resisting arrest for drunk driving. The policemen in the program seem smug and amused.

I head back to my room and sit on the bed, reading a government report from the late 1970s on the community, a document the province calls a "community area analysis." The Cree people in this area of harsh Boreal forest worked in 'task bands' that were often extended family units, reaping just enough plants and animals to survive. In summer when it was easier to get food, people gathered together into a seasonal band. "Self-discipline, respect for others and for the environment were prominent characteristics in pre-fur trade times," asserts the report. The first Hudson's Bay Company fur-trading post opened in 1825 here, "although records are vague." The post opened and closed frequently because of changing fashions in Europe, over-production of pelts, and depletion of fur-stocks. Inevitably, the local economy became tied to the booms and busts of the commercial fur trade.

In the early 20th century the band signed a treaty, best described in the passive voice of an official document:

> In return for relinquishing all rights to the land, certain compensatory measures were provided for them [the band]. Hunting and fishing rights were retained, subject to federal regulations. A reservation, supplying 160 acres of land for each family of five, was promised…. Five dollars was given to each man, woman and child at the signing of the Treaty. Thereafter, the Indian agent distributed $5.00 per person annually at the Hudson's Bay post….

The government's largesse under the treaty was not sufficient, but commercial fishing and guiding provided some jobs as an alternative to trapping starting in the 1940s. Families had to give up trapping if they wanted to live together and have their children in school for the full year. Then in mid-century came the new Indian Act of 1951, an "act respecting Indians" that was named with beautiful irony, since it's difficult to see how the act respected Indians in any way.

The provincial report notes dryly that "squeezing 200 years of technological and social change into approximately 25 years has not always been easy, or successful." The lack of ease and success for this community shows up better in the next documents I look at, which are photocopies of correspondence by United Church ministers who worked here between the 1950s and the 1970s. One minister left in 1972 before his term was up because he felt the community was unsafe for him and his family. In his correspondence he cites an RCMP report that listed the community as having the highest per capita crime rate in Canada in 1969-70. He describes a man who "burnt his home down in a drunken rage," "a most violent and viscious [sic] rape" of a young white teacher, other rapes in the community, and "continuing drunkenness and violence." His correspondents, church administrators in Winnipeg, thought he exaggerated the situation, but they too saw "signs of ... severe social breakdown."

I worry about getting everything done tomorrow, given how nothing runs on schedule here. I worry about how suspicious everyone seems, and whether that means this trip will in fact be worthless. In the bedside table someone has left a Nora Roberts novel about a woman kidnapped by savage Comanches in 1875. She is almost raped by one of them, but saved at the last moment by a half-white Indian whom she eventually marries. The man is reluctant and the heroine has to shoot near his head before he proposes. Why don't I sleep?

ELDER

My instructions from Chief Beardy were to be ready at 8:30 am. Paul would come by with his truck and he would show me around the community. Once again, I pace back and forth in the lobby of the motel. This time I pace around for only 10 minutes. I get in the truck with Paul and while I run him through my agenda, he ignores me and drives to the nursing station. He looks once at the over-cast sky and says "you might not fly outta here today." He is a large, stocky man who looks like he could move quickly if he had to. Now is not one of those times. He makes coffee and shuffles around the office with me hovering over his shoulder, hoping to communicate my awkward sense of urgency – I need to leave for the city today! I have a plane to catch, a book to write, deadlines to meet! For about half an hour I make myself relax and sit on the big sofa in the nursing station lounge with Paul and Owen. There is almost no talking. The phone rings in the distance. Then Paul stands up and says we will go to see an elder now – this was one of the things on my agenda that I thought he ignored.

The housing complex for elders is only a few hundred metres away but we drive over. As we park, Paul starts talking. He wants to know why I'm writing about their community and TB. I say that it's important for the outside world to know what's going on in places like this; I say that an invisible problem like TB in the north is one that just gets worse.

He listens quietly and then says "I hope that this book will not just benefit Dr. Hershfield, but will also be good for us here."

I feel a lump in my throat, simultaneously angry, guilty and sympathetic, and force myself to say "I hope the same thing," like the person who orders last in a restaurant and can't think of an original choice.

Inside the apartment on the edge of the complex is a small old man in a wheel chair with hands tightly clenched from arthritis. He speaks only Cree, so Paul acts as my translator. The old man's eyes are vivid and alert, and he has muscular arms. I give him a gift pouch of tobacco and ask permission to turn on my recorder. He says yes, and nods. Then he sends his grandson, who wears a Vince Carter jersey, out of the room. I ask the elder what he remembers about growing up. Paul repeats my question in Cree, and then the elder talks for a long time.

The elder says he was taught how to make his own living by hunting and fishing:

"I was active and that's how I stayed well. I never really got sick." He believes that he has arthritis because of the many years he had to work outside in the cold. "It was hard in the old days, but people were free. They didn't just stay in the community. They used to travel."

I ask if he remembers when Hudson's Bay closed their local trading post. He remembers the last time he took a fur to the Hudson's Bay post when he was 15. He is now 79, so the post closed about 1940. Then I ask him if he knew anyone who got TB.

Paul translates his answer: "People who got TB left for a long time. I don't know how TB came to be in our community. Maybe it came from the Hudson's Bay post or other visitors. Some people were affected and they went out for a long time."

The old man picks up his toast and chews while I ask my next question. Surprisingly, he has all his teeth. "What do you think are the most important problems in your community?" This time the elder pauses for what seems like a long time after the translation before he answers. Then he says:

"I feel that the land was taken away. When the treaties were made, we were told to stay in one area, not like before when we used to move freely to other areas and come back here in the summer time. The government promised it would look after us if we stayed in this community, and now I don't know if the promise was kept. Nowadays everything that the government is giving for the band is very limited. Housing is very limited, welfare is very limited, not too many people can make a good living on welfare! [He laughs.] Hardly anybody works nowadays. This year we hear there won't be anymore housing."

I also ask him about what the health problems are in his community. He says "what makes people sick now is too much junk food — potato chips, drinks. Now everything is full of sugar. The other thing is the alcohol and illegal drugs in the community."

"What about the young people," I ask. "What are your concerns about them?"

"You used to be taught when you were young how to make your own living. I sometimes wonder why these things are not taught at the school level – hunting, trapping, making a living from the land, that's what I would like to see, more teaching about our own lifestyle, making a living in a natural way. I know that the school has a different style of learning that the government wants, but they need to start teaching our traditions, our lifestyle, how to work together. I worry about the young people." This last statement has come in a few installments through Paul, and then there's another one: "Nowadays people don't want to walk, they just drive everywhere – riding everywhere on a snowmobile is not too healthy for the body. We used to walk around quite a bit."

The elder pauses much longer now and scratches his chin, and I start asking my next question. He starts laughing and says something in Cree, and I apologize, thinking I've interrupted. Then Paul laughs too. Paul can see I'm confused, and so he translates the last thing the elder just said: "I think maybe if you keep asking me questions we'll be here all day!"

I tell him we're almost done, but that I have one last question. "What should people in the south know about living in the north?"

"I don't know much about the south. People would feel different if they came up north. I think they would be very cold up here. Our land is beautiful and our water is drinkable. One time I was in the city but I didn't drink the tap water because I didn't trust it. There's too many people living in the south."

I shake hands with one of his arthritically twisted hands, and he has a surprisingly strong grip. He smiles and says he hopes we can talk again some time. Paul and I get back into his truck.

SCHOOL

We drive around to the other side of the lake where there is a small school for the kids who live on this side – the larger band-operated school is on the side of the lake where the nursing station is. This side of the lake features a motel that is apparently mostly a bootlegging front, and the RCMP station. The station is by far the most modern, solid-looking building in the community; maybe that United Church minister from the 1970s would have felt better when he saw this impressive structure.

When we pull up at the school there is a tall white-haired teacher yelling at a couple of kids to get inside and behave themselves. Paul and I are ushered into a large open classroom by the other teacher. The room is surrounded by whiteboards, brightly colored posters, musical instruments, and a few new computers. One of the boards has a series of exhortations urging the kids not to play with toy guns since violence is wrong. There are seven kids in a row on chairs in front of Jonathan, who has already started his presentation. He is down on the floor with two cut-out human figures.

Jonathan is explaining that tuberculosis is an old disease that goes back to ancient Egypt and the mummies. The last word seems a bit humorous to the kids. He explains that there are two kinds of tuberculosis: one kind is waking, and the other is sleeping. The waking kind can be spread when somebody coughs or sings or shouts, and somebody else breathes the germs in. He puts a cut-out picture of spraying particles in front of one of the figures' mouths on the floor. Jonathan says the sleeping kind can wake up later, and that's one of the reasons TB is a sneaky disease. He puts another graphic on one of the figures to stand for a TB germ, and talks about how the germ is like a hard-boiled egg, difficult to crack and get rid of.

Every couple of minutes Jonathan stops and asks the kids a question. They have to write their answers down on paper. He asks them now how TB is spread. The kid on the far right asks "how do you spell cough?" Jonathan spells it for him and the adults all grin at each other. When they read out their answers one of the girls thinks you can spread TB with plates and kissing. Jonathan says everybody's answer is "very very good," but actually TB can't be spread with plates or forks or kissing. Coughing is one way it spreads. Also "houses are better in Winnipeg" and so "bad air" in the northern houses makes people sick.

The kids are highly distractible until Jonathan pulls out a couple of x-rays. Then everybody snaps to attention and stares – one of the kids mutters "cool" under his breath. Jonathan uses the extra moments of concentration to talk about TB symptoms, and how TB is sneaky, making people think they have a bad cold or pneumonia instead of TB. Within five minutes he's talked about skin testing for TB, TB in the spine, how culturing TB is like cooking, and HIV. The kids know a lot more about TB than most grown-ups in Winnipeg do. The boy on the far right seems to know the most.

After the presentation lunch gets delivered in big plain white boxes from the local fishing lodge that doubles as a pizza parlour. The kids are ravenous and stop talking and playing to concentrate on the food. Most of the adults retreat into the teachers' lounge. The woman teacher says that the boy who sat on the right side away from us has a good reason to know about TB: his mother died of the disease last year. Jonathan has us all fill in a feedback form so he can improve his presentation: like nearly everyone I will meet who works on TB, he is unfailingly earnest and committed.

CHIEF BEARDY

After lunch at the school, Paul drops me off at the band office and announces that I'll need someone else to drive me around for the rest of the day. There's a long weekend coming up because the community shuts down for Aboriginal Justice Day, or J.J. Harper Memorial Day as they call it unofficially. Paul will be going to Thompson to shop.

I get ushered in by Chief Beardy and his Health Councillor almost right away. We sit down again at the long table with the orange plastic chairs, and this time they let me turn on my recorder. Chief Beardy wears large-lensed glasses from the 1980s with coke-bottle lenses, and he stares at me unblinkingly when he talks. He doesn't take off his coat but shows no sign of impatience. The councillor, named Dan, is playing with a thumb tack on the table, but says something every now and then that demonstrates his attentiveness. Chief Beardy tells me that the "employment rate" in the community is about 10%. Everyone else is on social assistance or old age pension. The few people who do have jobs work for the First Nation, the school, or the nursing station. On the other side of the lake there are a few jobs with Northern Stores and the RCMP. The lake once supported a commercial fishing business that employed a few families, but the stocks are depleted and transport costs are high. Trapping isn't viable anymore. The government report I read showed pretty clearly that the number of jobs in the community decreased as the population went up through the 1970s, and there are even more people now.

Given that there are so few jobs in the community, I ask what happens to young people when they finish grade nine, the last grade in the local school. Many of them go on to finish high school and post-secondary degrees in Brandon or Winnipeg, but then the band can't afford to hire them. So many of the best-educated young people end up living in the city.

Chief Beardy says that it is hard to live in a community like this. I ask Chief Beardy what people down south need to understand about communities like his. "The people in the south don't understand life in the north, the isolation part of it. It's very hard on the people, not only the cost of living, but living a healthy life. A lot of our people used to use traditional medicines and that seems to have gone. When I talked to an elder he said he was taking 15 different medications, and I said in the old days did you use those, and he said no. I said you elders seem to have lost a lot of our traditional ways, never passed them on to the younger people. I don't mean to sound negative but … the knowledge of the old days … is sort of gone."

I ask the Health Councillor, Dan, about housing in the community. Is it adequate? Dan says that it costs about $140,000 to build one house, including transporting materials here from the south. The band has a $1.1 million a year budget for capital projects to build houses, maintain the roads, and run community projects like the motel where I'm staying and the elders' home. After all these other projects, there is only about $600,000 left for building houses each year, so that means at most they can build five houses in one year. Then some of that money is lost to interest payments on Canada Mortgage and Housing Corporation (CMHC) loans, since they build some of the houses on credit from

CMHC. Dan says 120 houses are needed right now. So their capital program is in a perpetual and deepening deficit.

"What about overcrowded housing here?" I ask. Chief Beardy says "yes, we have that issue, and we have homeless people here as well in the community, so we try and get relatives to support them," which of course means multiple families in already-small houses. "So housing is a big issue here," he continues, "and not only here but in every First Nation in Canada."

"You know," I say, "that every TB expert in the world is going to tell you that overcrowded, badly ventilated houses, with people going in and out, visiting their friends and relatives, is a perfect way to spread TB."

Beardy looks pained, and he looks away for the first time. "Once we found out about TB we went after INAC [Indian and Northern Affairs] to get more money for housing. This year I'm going after them again." The chief then suggests that I should lobby the local head of FNIHB to get more housing money for the community. I nod gravely, feeling helpless. Eager to change the subject, I ask Beardy whether he envies the reserves near big Hydro developments who get cash and jobs, at least for a while. He says "I'd rather keep the land the way it is than take their money. I just need more housing money, that's all."

"What do you say to people in the south who think that too much money already goes to First Nations, given that you already get so many things free?"

Chief Beardy puts his weight on his elbows and leans towards me. "I hear people make comments about how we get free education, free housing. But they don't know how much we paid for those things. We paid with our culture, our languages, our traditional lifestyle, our land. When I talk to the elders about the treaty, they agreed to share the land and the resources, they agreed to *lend* the land to the other signatories. But when I read the treaty we gave up everything. We've paid over and over for *free* housing and education and healthcare. And it hurts me to see my people who were once strong now so dependent on government, eh. We have to go back to the old way of life. My mother says our lifestyle will come back. I believe her when I see all this mad cow and this bird flu. I think western civilization will turn to that Indian way of life that once was."

The sun has moved half way over the lake, and Dan stirs a bit beside me, but Chief Beardy is still talking. "My biggest concern about TB was that the leadership wasn't aware of the problem until we discovered it on our own, last September." This was when the nurse from FNIHB came in and did a presentation for Chief and Council about TB. Given the multiple programs and levels of government involved in dealing with TB for northern communities, it's hardly surprising that communication was less than perfect. Chief Beardy observes that "if we're going to work together, then there must be communication between leadership and the various health teams within the provincial and federal government." But he has not dropped his grievance, and feels that the health authorities did not take him and the band council seriously: "It's always been like that, there's that attitude of 'oh we know what's best for them eh, they don't know what they want or need.'"

The last thing we talk about is whether I should withhold the identity of their community. Chief Beardy says that his "biggest concern is that people on the outside may find out how bad the TB problem is, nurses or teachers or RCMP, and it could turn them off and they decide not to come here." So I promise not to name the community. "I'm not ashamed of the disease," says the chief. "Things are getting better rather than getting worse." This seems overly optimistic to me, but I don't live here, and so I stand up and shake hands with Chief Beardy and Dan.

HOUSING

"SINCE TB IS PRIMARILY SPREAD FROM PERSON TO PERSON THROUGH RESPIRATORY DROPLETS, IT IS LOGICAL TO ASSUME THAT POOR, OVERCROWDED HOUSING CONDITIONS WOULD INCREASE THE PROBABILITY OF TRANSMISSION. THE ASSOCIATION BETWEEN OVERCROWDED HOUSING AND TB INCIDENCE, PEDIATRIC TB, AND TB MORTALITY HAS LONG BEEN RECOGNIZED." – FROM *TUBERCULOSIS IN FIRST NATIONS COMMUNITIES*, 1999, A HEALTH CANADA DOCUMENT

I am back at the motel, waiting for my next ride. This time it's the community housing coordinator, Peter, who's coming. It occurs to me that almost no one here wears a watch. When Peter's half an hour late, I call the band office and ask for Dan, since the Chief is rarely available. I ask where Peter is, and Dan says "stay right there" and hangs up. Another 20 minutes pass. Finally one of the women at the motel feels sorry for me pacing the lobby and calls the band office, speaking rapidly in Cree. She says there's a trailer blocking the ice road across the lake, and Peter will be here soon. Sure enough, in 10 minutes he drives up in a bright red Chevrolet four by four.

We drive across the lake on what amounts to a multi-lane ice freeway with young pine trees stuck in snow banks to mark the road. When we pass a slow-moving vehicle it seems like the road is a mile wide. Peter drives very fast and confidently. He's much more talkative than the nursing station people and the politicians, who were all very suspicious. He tells me a story about a guy called Nine Lives. First Nine Lives got cancer, went to Winnipeg, and came back cured. Then he went back to his old job driving a road grader for the band. One day he was driving the grader across the lake near the end of February and the ice broke. Nine Lives was thrown through the window on the top side of the grader as it went down into the water, and so he avoided being trapped underneath. His flotation jacket brought him up smartly to the surface of the water, and from there he just hopped back onto the ice.

We drive to a large stand of houses scattered beside the lake and park in front of one particularly decrepit looking small house. There are 260 houses in the community, Peter says. According to his records, 160 of them need either replacement or major renovation. One of the big problems with a lot of the older houses is that they don't have HRVs – Heat Recovery Ventilators that circulate fresh air and prevent moisture from building up. Lots of the houses have mold problems, which is good news for TB germs.

We walk to the house we're parked in front of and Peter asks the family's permission to come in. The house has under 800 square feet of living area, but two families totalling seven people live here. The ceilings are buckling, and there are signs of mold around the woodstove's chimney. Definitely no HRVs here. Ashtrays overflow in the kitchen and living room. One of the bedrooms has blankets on the floor but no sign of beds. A pregnant young woman greets us in the living room where she is watching Maury Povich on a new Sony TV. I give her a gift pouch of tobacco, feeling intrusive and stupid. Peter introduces me as a "reporter from Winnipeg."

We drive up to another house, this one with plastic stapled on the windows and the paint peeling off. Peter says eight people live here in three bedrooms. In this house we just poke our heads in and say hello. The entry-way smells of fish and feces and is covered with graffiti instead of paint. Two German shepherd puppies are wrestling each other in the entrance. Back in the truck Peter tells me that one person who lived in the house died of TB a couple of years ago. Then we drive by one of the newer houses built with CMHC loans. Peter says these have five bedrooms and are occupied by bigger families or extended families.

I ask him how many of the houses have indoor plumbing. Peter says that 60% of the houses have running water, but only half of those have full plumbing, and the other half have holding tanks for drinking water and septic tanks for sewage. 40% have no running water.

Peter also tells me that the school was shut down for two years because of mold contamination and poor air quality. It stayed in use for a couple of years after an INAC inspection that found nothing wrong. But "people started getting sicker and sicker." The band brought in an environmental health specialist and that was when the school was finally closed for repairs. Taking out the mold and making it safe again cost half a million dollars, and the school was only 13 years old. "That was a good environment for TB," says Peter.

The sky is slightly overcast and I ask him if he thinks my flight will be cancelled. He says yes, definitely. But then that's what everyone says if you ask. They may be trying to scare me.

THE NORTHERN STORE

"WE WERE NEVER POOR BEFORE WESTERN CIVILIZATION CAME UP NORTH. WE WERE INDEPENDENT, SELF-GOVERNING. WE MOVED AROUND AND LIVED OFF THE LAND. THERE WAS NO SUCH THING AS STORE-BOUGHT FOOD. WE WERE RICH. PEOPLE WERE ALWAYS STRONG, THAT'S WHAT THEY TELL ME. THERE WAS NO DISEASE."
— CHIEF BEARDY

Peter drops me off at the Northern Store, which is within walking distance of the airport. The Chief and the nursing station people were all very keen on me seeing the Northern Store, mostly to look at the prices. The store is like a large corner grocery, but it also handles clothing, some electronics, and video rentals. There is lots of Wonder bread, a similar product called Northern Bread, very little produce, and huge stacks of Pepsi and RC Cola, which seem competitively priced by local standards. Tabloids are the only literature in evidence – this week's *Star* is headlined "Hollywood Sex Stunts," something that seems even more alien here than it does in Winnipeg.

The table below shows the prices of some common groceries at the Northern Store and a Winnipeg grocery store in the same week. Outside the Northern Store you could buy gasoline at $1.05 per litre, when it was .72 on the same day in Winnipeg.

Grocery Item	Price at the Northern Store	Price in Winnipeg grocery store
Maxwell House Original coffee, 1 Kg can	$12.19	$4.93
4 litres milk	$10.59	$3.15
Special K, 475 g. box	$7.49	$3.96
Cornflakes, 400 g. box	$5.79	$5.89 for 1.35 Kg
Pampers, 24 diapers	$18.49	$9.97
Lean ground beef	$6.81/kilogram	$3.70
chocolate pudding snack, 4 cups	$3.25	$1.77
bag of baby carrots	$4.29	$2.28
bag of celery	$5.99	$1.65

Welfare rates are adjusted slightly to account for the high cost of living in communities like this, but that doesn't mean it's easy to pay $10 for four litres of milk, or almost $20 for a box of Pampers. And you better be really committed to a balanced diet if you plan to follow it here.

THE AIRPORT AGAIN

It's about a 15-minute hike from the Northern Store to the airport. Leaning against the airport are five brand new mattresses and box springs that arrived yesterday. Now they appear to be abandoned in the snow beside the shipping area, which is open to the wind and too small to shelter anything bigger than a small box.

In spite of the spooky predictions about the weather, the plane arrives on time in the late afternoon. I board with Roy, the Health Canada psychologist who is still eager to talk about his book. Conversation is impossible in the noise. But it turns out I'll share his company a bit more today, because the plane is re-routed through another community where some extra passengers are stuck. This place has a real airport, a modern building with large windows, a bank of pay phones, vending machines, and employees playing Solitaire on computers.

On the first leg of the flight I am seated downwind from a man who has had a lot to drink. Roy was smart enough to sit up-wind of everyone. When we land the first time, I go to the nice modern washroom to fill a water bottle. In one of the stalls, the man who smelled like a still is now vomiting explosively into the toilet. When I get back on the plane he re-seats himself in the same place and looks like nothing has happened. He smells slightly less bad.

In Winnipeg I am standing outside the airline waiting for a cab when Roy hails me. He and his wife and their four children are there in a big green van. They drop me off on their way home. It seems like I've been far away, and for a long time.

7

WHO YOU DON'T SEE

"TUBERCULOSIS PRIMARILY AFFECTS THE KINDS OF PEOPLE WE DON'T LIKE."
— DR. GEORGE COMSTOCK, WORLD'S LEADING TB EPIDEMIOLOGIST

TB is a disease of opportunity whose most typical victim is someone socially disadvantaged, someone hard for most of us to see. This means that TB is also an unequal opportunity disease. Your odds of getting infected with TB are not determined by some democratically organized global lottery. Your racial background has nothing to do with it, although for many years medical researchers confused race with social conditions. Earl Hershfield routinely calls TB a "socioeconomic disease." Living in over-crowded housing, in badly ventilated rooms, being malnourished, having HIV, coming from a high incidence country – these are all factors that increase your odds of catching the disease. High incidence countries are easy to identify: think of a place that's poor, and the chances are they have a huge TB problem. Southeast Asia, most of Africa, the Indian sub-continent, China, these are some parts of the world where TB is rampant, and also places from where people immigrate to Canada and bring the disease with them.

So while anyone can win the TB lottery in theory – it is an infectious disease spread by breathing, after all – the odds are stacked in a very specific way. The most vulnerable populations in Canada are Aboriginal people, immigrants (Health Canada calls them "foreign-born"), street people, and the elderly. In 2001, the foreign-born made up 19% of the Canadian population, but accounted for 62% of all the reported TB cases. Aboriginal people born in Canada represent only 4% of the population, but they made up 18% of the TB reported in this country. 2001, the latest year for which national data's available, marks the first year that the proportion of Aboriginal TB cases was higher than the proportion of cases among Canadian-born non-Aboriginal people. Those of us who are not foreign-born, not Aboriginal, and not homeless form our own distinct demographic group of TB victims when we are over 65 years old. TB becomes more common in white men over the age of 75, likely because of damaged immune systems, although it's not understood why white men in particular are more vulnerable.

Infectious disease rates are measured per 100,000 people. In 2001, the Aboriginal rate of TB was 24.3, the foreign-born rate was 18.8, and the rate for the rest of us was 1.1. The national average was 5.5. Looked at regionally, Manitoba was at 10, and Nunavut had the highest rate with an astonishing 138.4 TB cases per 100,000 people. Manitoba's rate was high because we have a relatively large Aboriginal population, and Aboriginal people are still almost six times more likely to get TB than the average Canadian.

Disease statistics often tell stories if you're willing to listen. The story of TB statistics in Canada today is not too complicated. Immigrants often have a short-term problem with TB, but it's usually gone by the first Canadian-born generation. Aboriginal people, especially those in isolated areas, have an ongoing problem, something that should mark a blot on the social conscience of every Canadian. The same is true of street people, whom we ignore even more easily than First Nations communities in the north.

But the statistics don't tell us *why* things are this way. Earl says he thinks immigrants tend to comply with treatment and cooperate with the medical system because they desperately want Canadian citizenship and new lives; this is especially true when they are stuck in screening camps before they get here. Aboriginal people have no new life to look forward to – the problem is lack of change in a country that has robbed them of their land and is now apparently "compensating" them. Compliance and cooperation with doctors and nurses seems to vary based on people's circumstances and what they believe the future holds for them.

THIRD WORLD IN THE FIRST

I interviewed Phil Fontaine in January 2004 and we talked about the impact of tuberculosis on the Canadian Aboriginal community. Fontaine is the national chief of the Assembly of First Nations (AFN), the national organization of First Nations people in Canada. He has been active in Aboriginal politics since 1973, when he became chief of his own Sagkeeng First Nation in Manitoba at the age of 27. After two terms he worked for the federal government as a regional director in the Yukon, beginning his close and sometimes controversial ties with Ottawa Liberals. In 1991, he became Grand Chief of the Assembly of Manitoba Chiefs, and in 1997 he succeeded Ovide Mercredi as leader of the AFN. He was displaced for one term by Matthew Coon Come, whose contrasting style involved less diplomacy and more confrontation. Fontaine again took a federal appointment, this time as Chief Commissioner of the Indian Claims Commission. In 2003, he was elected once more as AFN national chief.

One of the reasons Fontaine is a national figure in Canada is because, in the early 1990s, he became the first Aboriginal leader to talk about sexual and physical abuse in the old Indian residential school system. What made Fontaine's speaking out so remarkable was that he talked about his own experience of abuse in a residential school. This was difficult for him and for his own community, but it led to a torrent of accusations and dredged up a piece of Canada's history that is truly shameful. The Catholic church, who ran 70% of the residential schools in Canada, continues to evade moral and financial responsibility for their actions, while the legacy of social destruction wrought by residential schools keeps playing itself out in every Aboriginal community in the country.

From early on in the history of residential schools, there were public health officials who saw clearly that they were a disaster. Dr. P.H. Bryce became the chief medical officer of the Department of Indian Affairs in 1904, and he wrote a report every year until 1914 about Indian residential schools on the prairies as breeding grounds for tuberculosis infection. His reports were never published or acted on, and in great frustration he published, in 1922, the year after he retired, a pamphlet called "The Story of a National Crime being an Appeal for Justice to the Indians of Canada." The appeal went mostly unheard: in 1948 Neil Walker, a superintendent for Indian Affairs in the prairie region, wrote "if I were appointed by the Dominion government for the express purpose of spreading TB, there is nothing finer in existence than the average Indian residential school."

The only significant thing that changed after Bryce's time was that Indians were now forcibly taken out of their communities when diagnosed with TB and taken to special "Indian hospitals." As we've seen earlier, the benefits of these hospitals and sanatoria were dubious except that infectious patients stopped spreading the disease in their communities. Nothing was done about the awful housing and poor diet in the residential schools that helped breed the TB bugs in the first place. Fontaine himself remembers an uncle who had a lung removed and then spent two or three years in a sanatorium. He also remembers kids disappearing from the residential school suddenly to be whisked off to a sanatorium somewhere.

Fontaine's office is in Ottawa, but he visits Winnipeg on a regular basis, often holding meetings at Winnipeg's only surviving railway hotel, the Fort Garry. We met in a large, airy room and it was easy to imagine an earlier era when white politicians used pleasant rooms like this to make non-consultative decisions for Fontaine's ancestors.

Fontaine believes that Canadians hold medicare as "sacrosanct," and put great emphasis on access and quality of care, but they also "don't appreciate that the community most compromised in terms of access to health care is First Nations people." Fontaine gave a few examples:

In southern Manitoba here you have two small communities where two new hospitals have been built recently, one for $40 million and another for $70 million and both hospitals are short of patients. These are communities with less than 1,500 people. You compare that to Island Lake, four communities, 10,000 people, nursing stations only, fly-in doctors, every woman that gives birth has to be flown in to Winnipeg. There are 24 dialysis machines in the province and only one of them in a First Nation community, yet the people that suffer most from diabetes are First Nations people.

Another example is what happens with x-ray technicians, who normally have to take a two year course to be licensed by provincial governments. X-ray services in nursing stations, on reserves, are done by people who have taken a two week course, and they're often former janitors. So the point I'm making here is that the health and safety of First Nations people has been severely compromised. There's not a word said by anyone when they talk about medicare or health as a priority that the interests they're advocating should include First Nations interests.

Fontaine thinks the reason for poor health in Aboriginal communities goes beyond the fact that many of them are remote, often far from major health facilities. He observed that the Indian Hospital in Pine Falls was closed by the government on the basis of an efficiency argument. The promise was that with only one hospital in the region everyone would get better health care. So Pine Falls General Hospital got bigger, they tore down the old Indian Hospital, and "our people have become sicker; there's no evidence that the health of our people improved." He pointed out that this was a community only a 90 minute drive from Winnipeg, so geographic isolation has not been a factor.

When it comes to TB, Fontaine was very aware of the fact that TB has re-emerged and that the numbers are actually increasing. He said, "It's well understood that TB flourishes in conditions of poverty, poor housing, and overcrowding," and noted that the high numbers of TB cases in Aboriginal communities "speaks volumes about the poverty of First Nations people."

Given the fact that many First Nations are in the process of taking over responsibility for their own health care, I asked Fontaine about the connection between self-government and health care. He said that the context is very important – "government has been an overwhelming force in our lives for a long time. For a long time they've decided how we should live." But the fact remains that "we're getting poorer, we're getting sicker, and we're becoming more dependent." "The way things are managed now doesn't work," said Fontaine, and so for him the long history of failed government intervention in Aboriginal affairs is the strongest argument for self-government.

Of course, there are skeptics when it comes to Aboriginal self-government. These are often the people who think all Canadians should be treated "equally" or refer contemptuously to the "Aboriginal industry,"[4] as if Canada's indigenous people had cooked up their present situation as some kind of scam. I asked Fontaine what he would say to people who claim that corrupt leadership is the real reason First Nations people have trouble with poverty and health. Fontaine was also willing to address the scandal at Sagkeeng, the reserve where he's from, where a substance abuse treatment centre allegedly misused federal funds:

> Well look at Hollinger, or Enron. That's corruption of the highest order, corruption in the white community, right. People have argued for the longest time, including some of our people, that corruption is rampant in our community. Well, what people ought to do is come forward with the damn evidence. The situation in Sagkeeng with the treatment centre was on the front page of the *National Post* every day for weeks, while a 100 million dollar tax break for Canadian corporations was buried in the business pages.

Fontaine went on to say that it's neither corrupt leadership nor the reserve system that are to blame: "indigenous people are the poorest people in all parts of the world," and they have no monopoly on corruption "nor do most of them (outside the US and Canada) have reserves." Fontaine doesn't bother trying to explain why Aboriginal people are poor, and it shouldn't really be necessary – when you steal people's land and destroy their traditional way of life, no one should be surprised that they end up needing government support. In terms of the link between poverty and health, Fontaine said this:

> It's obvious to us: poverty breeds ill health. The sickest group of people in Canada are First Nations people. We have the highest incidence of TB, diabetes, certain cancers, heart disease, the highest incidence of hospital care. By all of the indicators of poor health we beat the standard. If you look at the socioeconomic circumstances, Aboriginal people are poor. The auditor-general recently issued a report on the housing crisis in First Nations and successive governments have failed our people in dealing with this issue more effectively. High unemployment, poor success rates in terms of education, and all of that speaks about poverty. Canada promotes itself as the best country in the world – at one point Canada was at the top of the United Nations Human Development Index, and now we're at number eight. That tells us that the level of productivity in First Nations communities has dragged down Canada's standing. If that's going to be changed or

---

[4] See Robert Collins' use of this term in his recent book, *Prairie People, A Celebration of My Homeland.*

reversed, we're going to have to change the social and economic circumstances of Aboriginal people. It's that simple.

Indigenous people all over the world suffer from the combination of poverty and high rates of TB. Australia's indigenous people had a TB rate four times that of the general population in 2002, while American Indians and Alaskan Natives had TB rates six times the US average in 2000.

Canada's TB incidence in Aboriginal people has its own peculiar pattern: as a 1999 report of the Canadian Tuberculosis Committee put it, "the incidence of TB in the Aboriginal population has been shown to vary inversely with the time interval of contact with the European settlers, higher incidence rates occurring in those areas last exposed." This means that rates are highest in the north and on the prairies, and lowest in eastern Canada. When the elder I spoke to up north talked about how maybe TB had come to his community because of European visitors, he understood the problem's origin as well as any modern epidemiologist.

INTIMATE CONTACTS

Judy Riedel, who was a patient educator at the Respiratory Hospital in Winnipeg for almost 20 years, knows exactly how difficult it is to do contact investigation for patients from First Nations communities in the north. Many houses have 10 or 12 people living in them, and "there might be 30, 40 people dropping by a house in a day – so these are the contacts – it's absolutely amazing." Part of the detective work for the nurse doing contact tracing becomes looking at "treaty days, funerals, bingos, weddings, trying to figure out how people moved, relatives moving back and forth on reserves." Always it comes back to the question of whether the TB unit can locate the source case from which the infection is spreading.

Contact tracing is a difficult business in a First Nations community, and it is no easier with immigrants in the city. One nurse told me that "you have to keep being a detective," and at the same time "you really have to be sensitive to everybody's background." This is a difficult balance to achieve – while nurses get interpreters involved and try to be culturally sensitive, they also officially represent public health institutions, and TB is a reportable disease. This same nurse told me that "my belief was that their closest friend was the last name they'd give me; they were very protective of that person." But again, this nurse talked about informing the family and identifying the patient's worries to get appropriate referrals to social workers and psychologists. Diseases are often simpler than people's situations, but of course no one can separate the two.

Dr. Rey Pagtakhan, a federal member of Parliament since 1988, practised in the same hospital as Earl Hershfield in the early 1970s. He was a pediatric lung specialist, and later became a professor at the University of Manitoba's Faculty of Medicine. He spoke to me about the impact of TB on the Filipino Canadian community in Winnipeg, and one experience of his in particular. Pagtakhan first got involved in this case because a child whose family had recently immigrated from the Philippines was admitted to the hospital showing symptoms of TB on a chest x-ray. When this happens, doctors assume that the child was infected by an adult source. So the medical team carefully screened the parents and other family members for TB, and they all tested negative:

> I kept asking 'are there any visitors that may have come who were coughing?' So the answer from the parents was 'no.' But we said the infant must have been exposed to somebody. One day I was visiting and the grandmother was there. So I repeated the question. 'I'm told there have not been any visitors in the household. We are puzzled. We have x-rayed you, the parents, the older relatives that have come here, and nobody has tuberculosis. If we cannot trace that source, you and the other children could be infected. So I have to know. No visitors whatsoever?'

Then the grandmother admitted that there had been a visitor from the Philippines who had no visa. Pagtakhan assured her that he was a doctor, not an immigration officer, but that he had to deal with the medical issue. The visitor came in for an x-ray, and it turned out he was highly infectious with TB. His contacts also needed to be treated, including an RCMP officer who was investigating his immigration case. As doctors often do, Pagtakhan ended up being the visitor's advocate at the hospital. A visitor would normally have to pay for treatment, but neither he nor the family he was visiting could afford it.

The hospital readily agreed to do initial treatment, but then the visitor would have to go home to get the full year of drug therapy he needed. Who would pay for that? At this point Pagtakhan pointed out to Earl that it was a public health issue – if the man was not treated in Canada he would end up with incomplete treatment and infect more people in the Philippines. Earl was sympathetic to this position, and he agreed to provide the full year of treatment for the visitor at no charge. "How he did it, I guess," says Pagtakhan, "was the Medical Director's discretion."

"SPECIAL POPULATIONS" AND TB IN MANITOBA

Infectious disease specialists talk about "special populations" where TB is endemic in a specific part of the community. In Manitoba, Aboriginal people, immigrants, and the homeless are the special populations that bear the brunt of most of our TB. The problem is that these special populations are segregated enough from the rest of Manitoba citizens that their health problems seem invisible outside their own communities. That makes it hard for many of us to understand the challenges facing these groups related to geographic isolation, cultural displacement, and poverty. Dr. Beth Henning, who was medical officer of health in Sioux Lookout, Ontario in the 1990s, says TB in the Aboriginal community is all too easy to ignore for other Canadians:

> How easy it is for us white middle class people living down here in the south to ignore the problem. The numbers are small except when you look at them as a proportion in these small communities. It has everything to do with the social determinants of health: where they live; their access to all the things that keep people healthy including relationships, healthy communities, food choices, exercise, employment.

David Penman, who worked as a doctor with Indian Affairs in Inuvik from 1984 to 1988, talked about geographic isolation and how that creates problems for delivery of health care:

> You've got to recognize the dimensions of the problem. The population is very small, highly dispersed, but as Canadian citizens they're entitled to health care, and of course you have the overlay of special treaty commitments. The difficulty has been getting into these extremely small communities and detecting cases. This is very important because if they detect them it can prevent the development of cluster outbreaks.

Cluster outbreaks, where people in a small group infect each other with the same strain, are the mechanism that causes much of the TB among Aboriginal people in Manitoba. A recent master's thesis by Linda Olson[5] shows that a handful of isolated First Nations communities produce a large share of the province's TB cases every year. There isn't as much data on Aboriginal people in urban areas, or on those who do not have treaty status, but other evidence suggests that they too may experience cluster outbreaks related to inadequate housing. A 2004 report on Aboriginal housing issues released by the Institute of Urban Studies at the University of Winnipeg shows that over a two-year period, half of Aboriginal people who move to Winnipeg are unable to find affordable housing. They become what the study calls the "hidden homeless," living in overcrowded conditions with a series of friends and relatives. These are, of course, perfect conditions for a cluster outbreak of TB.

Immigrants face their own set of challenges related to TB, and their stress may not be obvious to more established Canadians, even if it should be. Many of these people are dealing not only with a new country, but also a new language, a new job or multiple jobs, and possibly separation from other family members. And of course this list does not include the often incredible hardship that immigrants have experienced before they got to Canada. These are precisely the

---

[5] *A Comparative Study on the Incidence of Tuberculosis Among Status Indians and Other Selected Groups in Manitoba, Canada,* University of Manitoba, 1999.

kinds of circumstances that break down immune systems and turn latent TB infection into active disease.

Since one of the biggest issues in TB control is compliance with a very difficult drug regimen and also preventing the spread of the disease when patients are contagious, healthcare workers need to be aware that immigrants, refugees and Aboriginal people may all have legitimate reasons for being suspicious of authority figures. Refugees may be used to only accepting something as an order if it involves physical force. And their problems in Canada are so numerous that taking pills after they already feel better might seem pretty trivial. Former patient educator Judy Riedel says that if hospital staff order a patient to wear a mask in the cafeteria, for example, they need to be aware that an immigrant may not take that order very seriously: "to us it's an important rule, it's infection control, but to them if you put it in the context of their whole life situation it may not seem that important."

One of the patterns common to nearly all immigrant cultures is close-knit family groups. Often extended families live together in crowded housing, pooling their money and resources so they can make it in the new world. When grandparents in an extended family find out that they may have given TB to their grandchildren, they are often terrified, partly out of guilt but also because they may be responsible for babysitting half a dozen children while the parents work. Family members who provide childcare often minimize their own side-effects from TB drugs so they can get home as quickly as possible. For them TB is a tragedy on a number of different levels: there's stigma associated with the disease, but also their labour is essential to the household economy.

Another issue for many immigrants is that they are setting aside as much money as they can to send back home to assist other family members. So a disruption of their ability to work is a problem not just for one person, but also for a whole extended family network. Sometimes it will delay or prevent other family members from joining them in Canada. In many ways healthcare workers adjust to the idea that immigrants are not going to be grateful that they've been diagnosed with TB. On the contrary, the diagnosis is what Riedel calls "a thorn in their sides."

STIGMA

Marian Roth, the nurse coordinator for some of Earl's ongoing research, says that "there is often a horrendous stigma about having TB" among immigrants, to the point that healthcare workers give permission to patients to say they have pneumonia, so they can avoid being shunned in their own communities and workplaces. Of course, contact investigation by its very nature makes complete secrecy impossible. Another nurse who works in ward H6, where TB patients are hospitalized in Winnipeg's Health Sciences Centre, told me that some patients simply refuse to believe their diagnoses – denial is their coping mechanism. The nursing staff won't argue with patients as long as they take their TB meds.

Roth talked about how patients think that having TB will reflect negatively on their hygienic practices, and will often go to extra lengths to clean up to avoid that perception. Riedel noted too that immigrants sometimes don't understand how the disease is spread. Just like Europeans did two centuries ago, people will sometimes throw away curtains and "practically sterilize all the clothing" of TB patients. Also, sometimes "couples didn't want to touch each other" for fear of spreading the infection. Riedel remembers spending a lot of time convincing a husband that his wife was no longer infectious and that they could, at a minimum, hold hands.

When immigrants are told that they likely brought the TB germ with them from their country of origin, they are often offended. Given their previous experiences with authority figures, they may not believe the explanation even if they understand it. They may also find it preposterous that they are asked to take medications that make them sick with side-effects for almost a year, when their friends back home took meds for one or two months and survived.

Judy Riedel says that "what the immigrant population worries about is that we're going to send them back to their country – they're terrified of losing their jobs, they don't have enough hours to have sick benefits, and they're worried about being shunned by their co-workers or even their own families."

Sometimes the diagnosis is more shameful than people can bear. Earl tells the story of an immigrant family being visited by their 10-year-old niece from back home. The girl felt sick and finally went to the hospital. She was diagnosed with tuberculous meningitis, a rare form of childhood TB that is nearly always fatal. The TB unit began treating her. A few weeks into the treatment, her uncle and aunt came in during visitors' hours and whisked her off to the airport. Before the authorities could intervene, she was on a plane flying back home. Earl says it's very likely she died, since her country has a very deficient TB control program and her family was too poor to pay for treatment.

In the Aboriginal population, Roth notes that "there's so much TB out there" that there is little stigma attached to the disease. HIV carries a lot of stigma, but "if you meet one person who's had TB likely half their family has had it," and "people in the community are aware of that." Strangely enough, the first experience of the south for some Aboriginal people from remote communities is triggered by their TB diagnoses. Roth talked about how difficult it is for Aboriginal people when they have to come south for a few weeks for TB treatment:

> When a case comes down here from an isolated northern reserve, a lot of them have never left the community. They're crying, they're lonesome for home. Even though TB is treatable and they won't be here long, when they have to be by themselves here it's really difficult for

them. They have the Aboriginal services here to visit them. Often times people are so lonely that family members come down to visit them.

STREET PEOPLE

Marian Roth, who's been Earl's senior research nurse for the last few years, says that if someone asks her at a party what she does, she replies "I'm a research nurse working with tuberculosis." The response is often "oh, I thought that was a disease of the poor," as if that meant the rest of us would somehow be insulated from such a contagion. That is not necessarily the case. In the early 1990s the south Point Douglas region in downtown Winnipeg had an average annual incidence of 474 cases per 100,000 people, roughly 47 times the national average. The middle class people from Winnipeg suburbs who worked in the area were definitely at increased risk.

People who live on the street, sleep on bridges or at homeless shelters are often amazingly tough and resourceful. They are also not likely to go to a doctor if they get sick, and it's very likely that they abuse alcohol or drugs. They are people like the Laurel and Hardy pair whose story I told in the prologue, walking around downtown Winnipeg with infectious TB. The disease can be spread in 15 minutes if conditions are right. Maybe a disease of the poor should concern us.

INVISIBLE HEALTH CARE

Early in 2004, the Manitoba Lung Association sends a team to do x-rays on some of the customers and staff of the McLaren Hotel. This is part of a contact investigation that started with a homeless person who had TB. It's early in the morning, and the bar lights are all off. The x-ray equipment is set up near the pool table, and traffic is brisk for the first half hour. Some of the people who get x-rays are staff members, others are patrons, some are just denizens of north Main Street. It's hard to see how any of them are denizens anywhere, actually. None of them look like they have a fixed address. In the darkness above the pool table hang two posters displaying Molson Ice girls who preside like bored goddesses. The Molson girls could be in a 1980s music video, but not the rest of this scene. This is health care most of us will never see.

There was a time when Main Street's McLaren Hotel was sophisticated enough to dub itself the "Hotel McLaren." You can see that high-toned version of its name on photos ranging from the 1930s to the '50s. In the 1960s my uncle, a horse-trader from Saskatchewan and a respectable businessman, used to stay here. The location was considered prime, and it's still across the street from the Centennial Concert Hall, home of the Winnipeg Symphony and the Manitoba Opera.

Al Harmacy, of the Manitoba Lung Association, tells me that his survey team does chest x-rays for TB at the McLaren Hotel every year. When I visit the

McLaren Hotel I notice a large sign in the lobby that says "Undesirables May Be Ejected". It is not clear exactly who management might consider undesirable. Rooms cost $30 with a shared bathroom, and $5 more gets the luxury of a private bath. Many of the patrons are from up north.

As you walk into the McLaren Hotel's bar from the lobby, the first thing you see at the opposite end of the large room is a shiny industrial-metal countertop. To the right of the bar is a raised bandstand. On both sides coming in are rows of Video Lottery Terminals. A man stands in front of one, propping himself up with one hand. He has an enormous belly stuffed in a plaid shirt and a bulbous nose poking out from his hunting cap. He keeps pressing a button on the VLT, expressionless. There were slot machines in hotels like this one back in the 1920s, positioned to steal from poor immigrants but not operated by the government.

In the bar there's a smell of piss and beer commingled in a way that even a Nobel Prize-winning chemist could not disentangle. Before prohibition this bar would have been called a "boozery". The room has high ceilings and a strange mixture of overhead lights and scone fixtures from a 1950s motel. On one side in front of the men's washroom is a Pioneer Laser jukebox with Nazareth, Elvis, the Rolling Stones, and a whole lot of country music: Pam Tillis, Marty Stuart, Dolly Parton, Garth Brooks. Right now the jukebox is playing George Jones' 1981 hit, "If Drinkin' Don't Kill Me (Her Memory Will)". Along the wall opposite the jukebox is the dance floor. Everyone here is working more on alcoholic suicide than remembrance of things past, and nobody's dancing.

THE REST OF US

Lee Reichman, of the National TB Center in New Jersey, believes that "we need to have some poster child die of TB – some high ranking government official, or a movie star." Even this wouldn't be enough to get real, concerted action on TB, he says. High-profile deaths from TB need to happen "continuously" to get public attention. Robert Marks, former controller and executive director of the Manitoba Lung Association, says something similar: "I don't think the public appreciate the problem that TB poses. I don't think they will until the white population start getting sick. It needs to get into River Heights." John Sbarbaro, a TB expert from Colorado, told me that 400 North American school children need to get multi-drug-resistant TB to get the disease back on the public's radar screen. "We need victims we can identify with," he said. Perhaps we need to try harder to identify with the victims we already have.

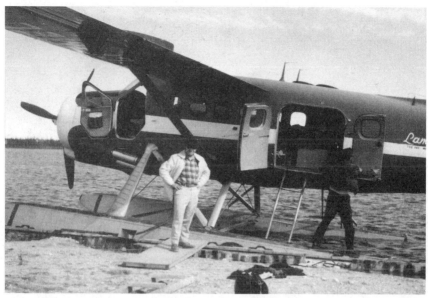

collection of Joann MacMorran

Earl Hershfield in front of airplane on North Knife Lake, Manitoba, 1968.

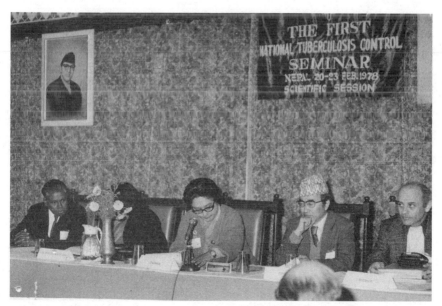

Earl Hershfield seated at right, guest of honour at the first National TB Control Seminar in Nepal, 1978.

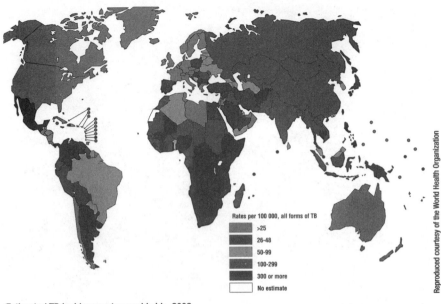

Rates per 100 000, all forms of TB

>25
26-48
50-99
100-299
300 or more
No estimate

Reproduced courtesy of the World Health Organization

Estimated TB incidence rates worldwide, 2002.

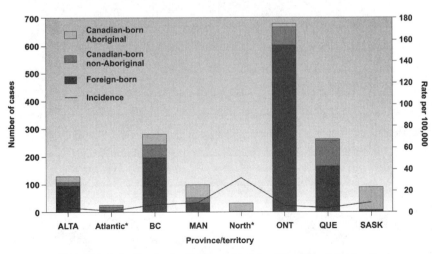

***"Atlantic" includes Nova Scotia, New Brunswick, Prince Edward Island, Newfoundland and Labrador. "North" includes Yukon, Northwest Territories, and Nunavut.

Source: *Tuberculosis in Canada — 2002,* Health Canada, 2004, reproduced with the permission of the Minister of Public Works and Government Services Canada

Distribution of Canadian TB cases by origin and incidence — provinces/territories, 2002.

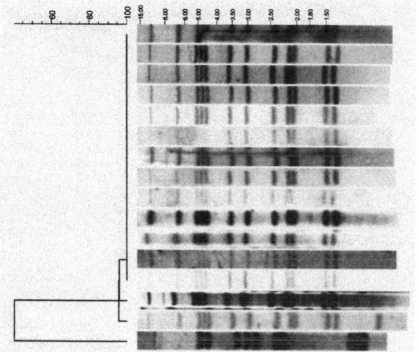

National Reference Centre for Mycobacteriology, at the Centre for Infectious Disease Prevention and Control, Winnipeg, 2004

Each of the horizontal bands is a DNA fingerprint of an individual's TB germ. The bracket lines on the left are called dendrograms and are used to compare DNA fingerprints from TB patients who come into close contact with each other. Vertical lines indicate a cluster of identical germs, demonstrating that the germs have the same source. The fingerprints here are of TB germs found in individuals from the northern community described in Chapter 6. The longest vertical bracket on the left shows that nearly all the fingerprints are identical, meaning that most of the TB in the community is the same specific strain, with the germ recycling through the population.

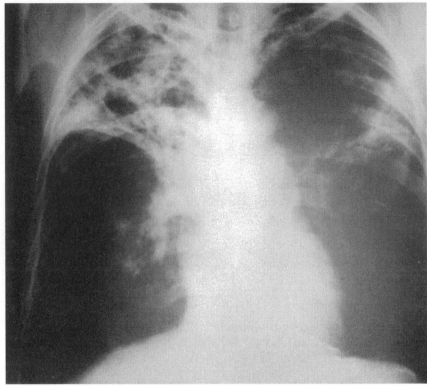

An x-ray of a patient diagnosed with advanced pulmonary tuberculosis in both lungs. Note the "caving formation" in the upper right lung (left side of photo).

Centers for Disease Control, Atlanta

Centers for Disease Control, Atlanta

Poster used all over the world to educate patients and healthcare workers about TB symptoms.

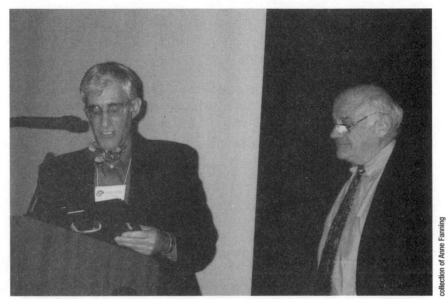

Lee Reichman presenting Earl Hershfield with the Distinguished Service Award of the International Union Against Tuberculosis and Lung Disease, North American Region, in Vancouver, 2000.

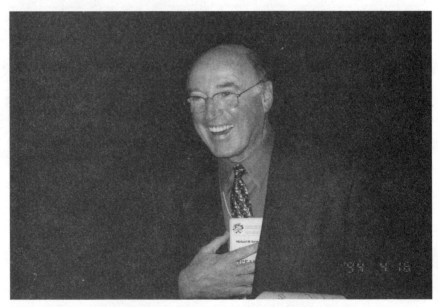

Michael Iseman, professor and tuberculosis surgeon at National Jewish Hospital in Denver.

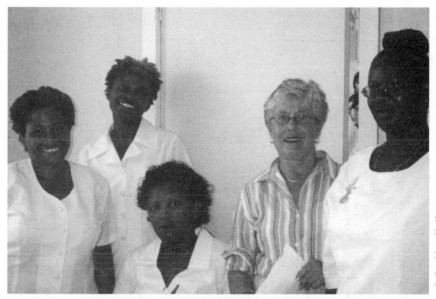

collection of Joann MacMorran

Joann MacMorran in Guyana with healthcare workers, 2004.

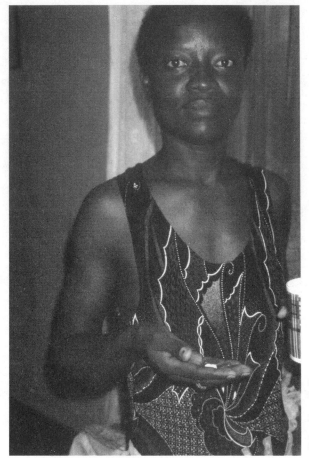

A Guyanese woman taking her TB pills, 2004.

collection of Joann MacMorran

8

MAKING CONNECTIONS

Energy, timing, and talent are all part of what make up a successful career, and Earl Hershfield has had all three in spades. When his career began in the 1960s, the first effective drug treatments for TB had just become available, and the first generation of Manitoba TB doctors were about to retire. But Manitoba needed new energy and leadership to set up a modern method for TB control after the sanatorium era ended with the closing of Ninette in 1972. Earl implemented modern drug regimens and new methods for TB control, just as other regional medical directors did in Canada and other countries at that time. As TB rates leveled off in the 1970s in Manitoba, and as the new, highly centralized program became established, Earl began to look for new challenges. He had remarkable, independent-minded people like Joann MacMorran in key positions, and much of the day-to-day work was now delegated. He still read all the x-rays and made recommendations on every individual case, something he would continue until his retirement from the directorship in 2003.

This chapter tells the story of how Earl became involved, first, in the national TB control scene in Canada, and then on the international stage, particularly with "the Union" – the International Union Against Tuberculosis and Lung Disease. Also discussed here is the story of how Earl demonstrated his passion for fair treatment of immigrants and refugees with his 20 years service on the Canadian government's Immigration Medical Review Board. Earl has spent a lifetime exporting his knowledge about TB control, and I outline just some of the work that he's done as well as some of the adventures he's had along the way. The chapter closes with a description of Earl's research work with TB drug trials and epidemiological studies.

GOING NATIONAL

In 1974, Earl was a member of the search committee for a new executive director for the Canadian Lung Association,[6] the body that is the national umbrella group for the ten provincial associations. In the past, this position had always been filled by a doctor, designated the "Medical Director." The search committee was having trouble finding someone in the Ottawa area, where the organization's offices were, and began to talk about having a Toronto doctor commute to Ottawa for two or three days a week. At this point Earl saw an opportunity. He suggested that, with all the direct flights from Winnipeg to Ottawa at that time, he could just as easily commute to Ottawa as a Torontonian could. He would be able to keep his job as Manitoba TB control director, but his responsibilities would be split between that and the directorship of the Canadian Lung Association. With the agreement of the other members, he resigned from the search committee and put his name forward for the position.

Earl was hired as executive director of the Canadian Lung Association in 1975. The search committee wanted someone who was a chest physician and not just a TB specialist, and who also had administrative experience. Earl fit that profile. But he was not prepared to move to Ottawa "for a variety of personal reasons." One of them was that Ottawa just wasn't any fun in those days: "It was a small town and they rolled up the sidewalks at seven o'clock and hardly had any restaurants."

After being hired in 1975, Earl cleared his desk at home in Winnipeg and began the new job January 1, 1976. He spent part of most weeks in Ottawa, and was available and in contact with Ottawa by telephone full time. He says now that his job would have been much easier if he'd had e-mail and a cell phone. However, he was ably assisted by the associate executive director, Hubert Drouin, who worked full time in the Ottawa office running the administrative affairs of the Association. Some of the provinces weren't happy with this arrangement, but Earl was characteristically more interested in implementing his vision than in pleasing everyone. The staff had no problem working with Earl – Drouin says "the distance between Ottawa and Winnipeg didn't seem to exist because he was so supportive of the staff," and also that he was "very easy to communicate with." Once again Earl was finding a way to get things done. Drouin says that "communications were as frequent as necessary."

One of the things that Earl initiated was changing the national organization's name from Canadian Tuberculosis and Respiratory Disease Association to Canadian Lung Association, a change that came about after much discussion at a 1977 meeting in Moncton, New Brunswick. The idea of a bunch of doctors and administrators fighting about their organization's name might seem a bit esoteric, but this was a very important issue. For the traditionalists, the word "tuberculosis"

---

[6] It was then called the Canadian Tuberculosis and Respiratory Disease Association.

could never be taken out of the name because that was the disease which the organization had been created to fight. Part of the difficulty with the name change, too, was certainly the weight of tradition. The organization goes back to the time when Sir Robert Borden, Canada's prime minister during the First World War, was "secretary" to the association, a position that amounted to what would later be called "executive director."

However, Hubert Drouin, who was the administrative head of the Canadian Lung Association from 1971 to 1978, says that "ultimately tuberculosis was not a word that was on the minds of younger people." So one issue was simply public visibility; for an organization dependent on an annual fundraising campaign – Christmas Seals – the name of the organization had to make sense to the general public who would be asked to give. The generation that had suffered with tuberculosis was getting older, and younger people benefited so much from the lower rates of the disease in Canada that they no longer considered it important.

Other than fundraising, public relations, and educational efforts, there was a much simpler reason for the name change: the organization was broadening its activities to include lung diseases other than tuberculosis. With TB in decline, the organization had to tackle new diseases and change the name, or, as Earl says, "we would have disappeared." During his tenure, Earl hired experts in asthma and COPD, or chronic obstructive pulmonary disease, which is mostly caused by smoking. Part of Earl's responsibility as well was to be involved with the Canadian Thoracic Society, which is the medical arm of the Canadian Lung Association. This organization was also becoming more involved with lung disease in general rather than focusing almost exclusively on tuberculosis, as they had in the past. The reason for the change in focus was because by 1975 almost all the TB specialist doctors had either retired or died, and the Thoracic Society became an association of respiratory disease doctors.

The next item on Earl's agenda was to convince the provincial organizations that they too should modernize their names and continue to broaden their focus. In Manitoba what is now known as the Lung Association was called the Sanatorium Board until 1975, and Saskatchewan retained the name Saskatchewan Anti-Tuberculosis League through Earl's tenure with the Canadian Lung Association. Alberta's provincial organization had already changed its name in 1968 from the Alberta Tuberculosis Association to the Alberta Tuberculosis and Respiratory Disease Association. Most of the provinces were led by people who had personalities as strong as Earl's, and besides this was Canada – fights between the regions and anything based in Ottawa are bred in the bone. Saskatchewan ended up holding on to its old name until the 1990s.

As with his work in Manitoba, Earl was the right person for a time of change. Drouin believes that the changes Earl initiated would likely have taken place regardless of who led the organization, "but they might not have turned out so well." In terms of Earl's management style, Drouin says he was very open and direct. He had no problem with allowing debate on issues, even if that debate sometimes resembled hand-to-hand combat. Earl was good at getting consensus on difficult issues, and you never had to guess where he stood on a particular issue: "You get what you see with Earl, he's very up-front."

Earl's style with the staff was less formal than what they had been used to with the old regime. They would kid him about "blowing in from Winnipeg" with his big fur coat and boots, and he was "a great kidder, fun to work with." One year when the annual meeting was held in Winnipeg, Earl kept the staff company while they waited for their flight back to Ottawa.

Earl became very familiar with both the Winnipeg and the Ottawa airports in the 1970s, continuing to juggle his two very demanding jobs. He stayed on as executive director of the Canadian Lung Association until 1982, when there began to be pressure to move to Ottawa full time. "I had to move there or I had to get out," as Earl puts it, and his family life still revolved around Winnipeg. As well, by 1982, his international work was keeping him on the road more and more.

INVOLVEMENT WITH THE UNION

Having launched his national career, it was inevitable that Earl would begin looking at the rest of the world. In a sense, all he was doing was following the patients; then as now, TB was rampant in the developing world, and more or less under control in North America and Europe. The prime vehicle for Earl's international involvement in TB was the International Union Against Tuberculosis and Lung Disease (IUATLD), in which he had a voting membership as executive director of the Canadian Lung Association.

"The Union," as TB people call the IUATLD, is, along with the World Health Organization, the most important international body involved in TB control. Dr. Don Enarson, a Canadian who now is the Scientific Director for the Union, says that the Union's role is akin to that of the university public health department, but at an international level. In other words where university public health departments advise local governments on health policy, the Union advises the World Health Organization on policy with respect to tuberculosis and lung disease. He says "I see our job as pioneering things, testing things out, showing the way, questioning existing policies, and teaching."

So Earl inherited a membership in the Union, and that helped spark his interest in working internationally on TB control. The Canadian Lung Association's history with the Union went back to 1961, when the Union's annual meeting was held in Toronto. Dr. Edward O'Brien, the longtime head of the Ontario TB Association, suggested that the Canadian Lung Association and Canada become involved in the "Mutual Assistance Program" of the Union. This program provided financial aid primarily to voluntary TB health organizations in under-developed countries. The rationale was that in poor countries it was essential to get local volunteers for indigenous TB programs, to help those programs with providing education and getting people to take their medications.

As a result of O'Brien's leadership, Canada was soon directly involved in TB control programs in a number of countries concentrated in Asia. The Canadian Lung Association's mandate now included international aid. Assistance initially focused on developing the voluntary sector in these countries, and later for projects in countries that lacked an active voluntary TB organization. One project that began in the 1960s in Sri Lanka involved traveling seminars and provision of a van and scooters for volunteer health workers. Also in the 1960s in Malaysia there was a Mutual Assistance program that piloted projects in three districts using officials and volunteers in TB case-finding and case management.

Funding at first came from a special levy of one percent on the Christmas Seal Campaigns of the provincial lung associations. This was controversial, since many people felt that money raised in Canada should be spent here. By the mid-1960s the pressure eased when the Canadian International Development Agency (CIDA), an arm of the Canadian government, started providing matching funding on a project-by-project basis.

When Earl took over the Canadian Lung Association in 1976 the organization's involvement in the Mutual Assistance Program had begun to wane. Earl says "I fought battle after battle to get the Canadians to keep being interested in tuberculosis control outside North America." Earl's interest in immigrants and refugees was tied to a pragmatic sense that "you can't do TB control without working in poorly developed, high-incidence countries, because those people come to Canada." In other words, TB problems in other countries turn into our problems when people immigrate to Canada.

INNOCENT AMERICANS

Michael Iseman of the Denver Jewish Hospital says that "Earl and Canadian physicians have had more of a sense of global attachment than US doctors have." He characterizes American doctors as "parochial" and facing a lot of pressures in their immediate community, whereas in Canada there is "an expectation of outreach." Over many years of seeing Earl at conferences and committee meetings with the Union and the American Thoracic Society, Iseman says

> As long as I remember, Earl was the conscience of those of us who practiced TB in North America, making us aware of the immense burden abroad. In addition to serving our own communities we had a moral and professional obligation to get involved with the big world out there where there was so much TB and so few assets. If you ask me what stands out about Earl it would be his awareness of that and his prodding of us here in North America to look outward.

Earl sees one of his major contributions in the Union being that he got a new generation of American doctors engaged with international tuberculosis. In the 1970s and '80s tuberculosis was perceived within the medical profession as a dying disease (because it was fast disappearing at that time in North America), and so there was a vacuum where there should have been activity. Earl says "there were hardly any lung doctors interested in public health and international studies." He was amongst a handful of maybe a dozen people who were interested, mostly Europeans with a sprinkling of Canadians and Americans. Certain European countries, like the Dutch, the Norwegians, and the Swiss, were putting a lot of money into the Union, but that was not the case with North American governments.

One of the avenues Earl used to drum up more interest with Americans was through the American Lung Association, with whom he had good relations. Earl believes that the Canadian Thoracic Society had better meetings and superior scientific papers than the American society in the 1970s and early '80s. The Americans at the time were "insular, not interested in the world around them." But the new generation of doctors in the society, Earl thinks, was "more liberal-minded than their predecessors." He attributes this to the fact that they were university people, "not earning seven figures," and therefore more liberal and outward-looking.

NORTH AMERICAN CHAPTER OF THE UNION

In 1979, Earl made his most visible contribution to the Union when he co-founded, along with Dr. Jim Kieran and Dr. Lee Reichman, a North American chapter of the Union. It may seem strange that there hadn't always been a North American chapter. However, when the Union was originally established in 1920, it was an association of national organizations that increasingly evolved into regional bodies. The organization was based in Paris and was dominated by the European region. North America's incidence of TB had been relatively low even in the 1940s, when the Union was revived after the war, and so there was a feeling that North Americans didn't really have much to say about TB anyway. Dr. Philip Hopewell, who later became president of the Union's North American region, notes the odd fact that "North Americans and particularly the American Lung Association had always been major contributors to the operating costs of the Union, yet there was not really a voice that was listened to from the North American region."

What had happened was this: the term of the American representative on the Union executive expired in 1978, and the previous Canadian representative had retired in 1975. So in 1979, North America was sending money to the Union but getting no chance to influence policy. What Earl, Lee Reichman, and Jim Kieran realized in 1979 was that each region of the Union automatically got a representative on the executive. So the three of them got together at a hotel bar during a conference and organized a North American region. They elected Lee Reichman as chair and then had him appointed to the Union's executive since he was now in charge of an official region. Until 1996, the region was just a political convenience, and then North America decided to have its own scientific meeting. These meetings are now the largest and most well-reputed scientific meetings devoted exclusively to tuberculosis in English anywhere in the world. Hopewell says that Earl "had a good understanding of the politics of the Union and of the international scene of tuberculosis control," which was no doubt true. He was about to learn more, though.

FOREIGN STYLES AT THE UNION

Meetings at the Union were not run the way Earl was accustomed to back home. Americans and Canadians expected people to move and second motions, and a chair to keep order and make sure outcomes were logical and efficient. The Europeans and other non-North Americans on Union committees had a different style. Earl remembers being in Paris at a Union meeting and discussing the details of a TB treatment program. A lot of different people spoke and a lot of them made motions – there were twelve motions in all. A number of them overlapped and contradicted each other. The committee voted, and the two motions that passed were mutually contradictory. Here's Earl's account:

> Everybody had an opinion, and everybody's opinion was slightly different. It had to do with language, translation, it had to do with why them and not me, so that particular meeting had no tangible outcome except interestingly enough by osmosis things eventually got done. Not the way I'd learned to do things, but people began to understand what should be done, and so that to me was an eye-opener.

Earl also became good friends with the vice-president of Mali, who was also physician to the king, and the possessor of a highly ambiguous style. Earl says "he was a very bright guy, but he always had a position that was, 'well, let's see, let's think about this.'" For a blunt, pragmatic Canadian, this was a new experience.

Another issue that resurfaced for Earl was changing the organization's name. It had always been the International Union Against Tuberculosis. This time Earl, along with his American and Dutch counterparts on the executive committee, wanted to stick with tradition. They thought that tuberculosis control needed to be the top priority of the Union, and changing the name would weaken their focus on TB. Many of the developing nations were represented on the executive, and their view was that it was old-fashioned and backwards not to include "lung disease" in the organization's name. Earl remembers it as a "highly charged" meeting. His faction lost the vote, but he hasn't changed his mind: he still thinks that the Union needed to concentrate its resources on tuberculosis.

TB DIPLOMACY IN CHINA

One of Earl's accomplishments in the Union was re-establishing China as a member, an important step because China had, and still has, a major TB problem. Earl was the first person to officially contact China about rejoining the Union, where their membership had been taken up by Taiwan since 1948. He visited China in 1981 with Manitoba politician Sidney Spivak. The Union arranged for the head of the TB Association in China, Dr. Guan-qing Kan, to meet Earl at a train station in Beijing. Earl became good friends with Kan, but because of political issues it would still take five years before China rejoined the Union.

Before Earl's intervention, the Union had been carrying on its careful style, leaving surreptitious messages for Chinese delegates at international meetings, or buttonholing delegates in the hallway. But nothing official happened. The rub was that China wanted to enter on the condition that Taiwan's membership would then be "discussed" and possibly abrogated. China considered then, as they do now, that Taiwan should not be independent from the mainland. After Earl's meeting with Kan, Earl ended up siding with Russia and Cuba in supporting China's bid for re-entry into the Union – it was going to be the only way to get modern TB treatment to millions of Chinese in the short term. The Americans and Europeans were strongly opposed, since for them this was a geopolitical issue rather than one about health policy.

For Earl this was once again a pragmatic issue – millions of Chinese suffered with TB, many more than in Taiwan, and he was willing to make a political compromise because he saw the health issue as more important. Earl remembers "yelling and screaming" at meetings about this issue. His side eventually won, and China became a member of the Union again by 1986. Taiwan was never ejected, but held a separate membership from China.

OH CANADA

In 1980, the Canadian and American Lung Associations held their second combined meeting in Washington D.C. The hotel where the conference was held was still under repair and rain was leaking through the roof in the hall during the opening ceremony. At the ceremony's official dinner, a smart-looking band of US marines marched up onto the stage with the American and Canadian flags. The Canadian flag, though, was upside down. They then played the "Stars and Stripes" and marched briskly off the stage. Earl walked over to the chair and whispered to him "how about the Canadian national anthem getting played?" The chair signaled an aide, the marines marched back in, and they played "Oh Canada" with the maple leaf still pointing downwards.

Earl's American colleagues all talk about his sense of pride and identity as a Canadian. Philip Hopewell says that "Earl is distinctively Canadian. He always made it very clear that Canada was different." Through the 1980s Earl was what he calls the "token Canadian" on many professional committees, and he made sure the Americans understood that he had a distinctively Canadian point of view. What that meant for Earl, among other things, was that he always put a higher priority on public health policy than on American foreign policy. If that meant offending some Americans by voting with Russia and Cuba sometimes, that was OK. It also meant that Earl was not always going to adopt the latest approach in Canada just because it was being pioneered in the US. For example, John Sbarbaro of the University of Colorado, who has known Earl for his whole career, describes him as a "challenging conservative; Earl would say 'I'll go so far, and I love to argue with you, but I'm not sure we can implement it in Canada at this time.'" This cautious approach to change served Earl well in his Canadian work.

In 2000, Earl became the first recipient of the Union's distinguished service award for the North American region. Earl had served as Secretary-General of the region from 1979 to 1992. Among other things, the award recognized Earl's work as Director of the Union's Mutual Assistance program from 1976 to 1985.

GOING ABROAD

Earl resigned from his position as executive director of the Canadian Lung Association in 1982, but he kept right on going with his international work through the Union. The first country in which he had a major involvement was Bangladesh, where the Canadian Lung Association and the Union planned to run a large vaccination trial, giving everyone under the age of 16 a BCG vaccination over a four year period and monitoring the prevention outcome. BCG's effectiveness had been questioned for some time by experts in the United States, but a lot of people in the field still wanted to conduct research.

This project would have been one of the largest modern field trials of BCG ever conducted, but unfortunately it was cut short by political upheaval. Earl went to Bangladesh in 1981 and stayed in the exact Chittagong hotel where a coup d'état was staged and the president assassinated. The new government, led by General Muhammad Manzur Ahmed, promptly kicked out all foreigners the day after the coup, including Earl. About two-thirds of the BCG vaccinations were complete at this point, but what was supposed to be a long-term project was instead aborted early.

This was to be the first of a number of times Earl had experiences that resembled the British novelist Graham Greene's, who seemed to always be in the middle of a revolution. Earl tells this story about another trip to Bangladesh:

> We went on what had been an English river boat with the Minister of Health, and he had three armed guards. We went into a town that had lots of TB. The guards had their bayonets fixed and were holding the crowd back. These are the adventures you get into if you do this kind of work.

Starting in 1978, and continuing through the 1980s Earl was also involved in Nepal. There he helped set up the Nepal TB Association and tried to convince the government to run a national TB program. As with most governments, and not just in the developing world, there wasn't much enthusiasm for a national TB control program. Earl worked with groups who were already in Nepal, almost all of whom were Christian missionaries except for the British Nepal Medical Trust, the Edmund Hillary Trust, and a few others.

Earl's experience in Nepal convinced him more strongly than ever of the importance of having a nationally co-ordinated TB program. What the missionaries did in Nepal was they set up small nursing stations all over the country. The catchment area for these stations was the limit that people will generally walk to receive healthcare, which research has shown to be about nine kilometres. So of course TB and other diseases were treated in a roughly nine kilometre zone around each nursing station. But between these zones, disease of all kinds was rampant. Especially for an infectious disease like tuberculosis, this regionally fragmented approach could mean that health workers just put out a local fire that continued to rage just around the corner and returned with greater ferocity every year. Earl says, "maybe this is a harsh way to say it, but unless there's a national program and national control of health, what you're doing doesn't really matter."

The aim of the Nepal TB Association was to put together all of the fragmented efforts into one national program, and also influence the government to fund it. For a while, the Nepal TB Association ran a hospital that was the only Nepali hospital treating TB, but it too was limited in its ability to reach across the whole country. The funding came from Canada and a few other donors. However, the Mutual Assistance Program provided funding to strengthen the association. They contributed to the salary of an executive director, ran two national seminars, and helped negotiate with the government and the World Health Organization for funding. Earl was heavily involved in building up the Nepal TB Association. After many years of effort by local people and international consultants, Nepal does now have a national program and declining TB rates.

The purpose of all of Earl's work with TB associations was "to make them strong so then they could advocate with their governments to fund national tuberculosis programs." In addition to his work in Nepal, Earl has also worked in Bangkok and Singapore with their TB associations. Earl has been a member of a Singapore International TB Advisory Board since 1990, and made a return visit to Thailand in the mid-90s.

IMMIGRANTS AND TB

Beth Henning tells this story about a Canadian meeting of regional TB control directors held in the 1990s. Someone had gotten up and said one of the biggest problems with TB control "was immigrants, and maybe we should just tighten up and not let anybody in." Henning at the time was the Medical Officer of Health for Sioux Lookout in Ontario, an area the size of France with 28 First Nations communities riddled with TB. Earl got up and said "I'm from a long line of immigrants." Beth reports him pointing at the person who'd suggested excluding immigrants with TB and saying:

> If you're not an immigrant your parents or your parents' parents were, and you're going to tell me that we're going to deny sick people the right to a new life? Why do they have tuberculosis? Why are they looking for a new place to live? If they're sick, bring them over, we'll treat them. This is not an insurmountable problem. This country was built on immigrants. Why would you deny people a life?

Henning describes Earl as simply shaming everyone. He was not willing to let people act in a way he believed was wrong. Earl remembers the same meeting. He says he spoke about how, as a son of immigrants, he could not exclude TB patients "because this is not my land; it is my country, but it's not just mine." Earl jokes about how maybe Torontonians and Americans assume ownership of their country, but he sees himself as privileged to live in Canada and eager to share that good luck with those who come to this country like his parents did, as immigrants and refugees.

Earl's most significant involvement with immigrants and tuberculosis began in 1978, when he joined the Immigration Medical Review Board, which at the time was part of Health Canada. The Review Board started largely because the Canadian government brought in the Immigration Act of 1976 and needed regulations on medical issues written into the Act, and also advice on individual cases. The doctor who was in charge set up an advisory committee on the medical aspects of immigration. Earl joined in his capacity as executive director of the Canadian Lung Association. By 1981, an unworkable 40-person committee got whittled down to 10, with specialists in psychiatry, infectious diseases, cardiology and so on. Earl was the designated TB expert.

Brian Gushulak, Medical Director for Citizenship and Immigration, sums up Earl's contributions on immigration and TB like this:

> Earl became the primary source of reference for TB and immigration for nearly 20 years in Canada. His role was to be a mentor, standard-bearer, and provocateur. He always focused on the importance of dealing with the disease and immigration in a humanitarian way.

During his early days with the Review Board, Earl wrote the new regulations for TB that became part of the Immigration Act. These changes to medical screening rules that he introduced represented a large shift in policy. They were designed to facilitate more efficient processing of immigrants with TB infection.

The new regulations were in turn approved by the Canadian TB group, mostly composed of regional TB control directors. The new regulations then became part of the Act with some minor revisions.

The new Immigration Act changed a lot of things in 1976. One of them was that it opened Canada to increased Asian immigration as European immigration continued to drop. With the end of the Vietnam war, there was a large number of displaced Vietnamese people who needed somewhere to go. Earl had already become deeply involved with southeast Asia through the Mutual Assistance Program. So now it would be a logical consequence for Earl to become involved with southeast Asian refugees and their problems with TB.

By the late 1970s, the Immigration Medical Review Board was confronted with the issue of TB primarily because refugees from Vietnam, Laos and Cambodia were being held in camps all over southeast Asia for long periods of time. They were processed to come to Canada but if a suspicious chest x-ray or other test that indicated TB, they weren't allowed to emigrate. So people who wanted to come to Canada were piling up in these camps, some of them on the Vietnamese border, and others in Singapore, Hong Kong, and Thailand. Earl was commissioned by the Canadian government to visit the camps and write a report with recommendations on how to clear the backlog of refugees with suspected TB problems.

The camps in countries Earl visited for his report were border camps of over-land refugees. These refugees were disease-ridden and had suffered terribly with malaria, diarrhea, and TB. One camp Earl visited was near the border between Vietnam and Laos. Officials from Canada, the US, and Australia were in the camp interviewing refugees as part of deciding whom to admit. Earl spent his time observing how medical tests were analyzed and interviewing people. He remembers a lot of 12 hour jeep rides over bumpy roads and his own bouts with diarrhea.

Earl's report featured a number of illustrative cases to bolster his recommendations for more streamlined TB screening. One man was delayed in this refugee camp for years together with eight members of his extended family because the authorities thought he had drug-resistant TB. Finally the man hanged himself, believing that he was a burden to his family and ruining their lives. Earl suspects that the whole case may have rested on a mistake in the lab, although it was impossible to prove that. Earl's report recommended better medical screening and treatment procedures so that refugees in camps like this would be processed more quickly and thus treated more humanely.

FIGHTS ABOUT POLICY

The routine business of the Medical Immigration Review Board, which Earl sat on from 1978 until 2001, was dealing with individual case review for immigrants who had medical issues that were difficult to make decisions about. The Review Board also did research to see that current policy was working and recommended immigration policies with respect to medical screening. Over time fewer individual cases had to be considered because previous ones formed precedents. As a result, the Review Board had time for an increasing number of policy recommendations.

This is where the frustration set in for Earl and some of his colleagues on the Review Board. The government nearly always accepted case-by-case recommendations while nearly always rejecting policy advice, even when the policy was a logical outgrowth of precedent already established by the Review Board's individual recommendations. Dr. Jay Keystone, a tropical disease specialist who served on the Review Board with Earl, says that "once we began looking at policy issues there was a lot of patting on the head and 'thank you, you're doing a wonderful job,' but nothing changed."

In the meantime, discussion of individual cases was often hot and polarized. Earl says "there were angry fights, really mad fights, because people were now baring their inner souls." Keystone remembers that Earl "would always give the immigrant the benefit of the doubt." Earl says that he argued "vehemently and loudly" on issues that he felt were "controlled by right wing conservatives who were anti-immigration." For Earl, these arguments were not simply professional discussions conducted in the passive voice, but deeply personal and emotional:

> I used to say 'if I weren't in Canada, where would I be? Probably killed in the Holocaust.' As a Jew, my parents, my ancestors have been wandering the earth, so I'm certainly not going to stand in the way of a legitimate Geneva Convention refugee, just because the colour of his skin is different, he doesn't speak English or French, or he has a medical condition that can be easily treated.

Earl was also one of the first people on the Review Board to favour admitting immigrants who tested positive for HIV, something that eventually became Canadian policy. He remembers the only other vote supporting the admission of HIV-positive individuals coming from someone he saw as right wing, and whose rationale was different than his. Keystone comments that "Earl often swung the board to his side, because he did have a sense of what was right and wrong as opposed to what went by the book." So for all his willingness to stand alone on a position, Earl did convince a majority of his colleagues at least some of the time. Every year the Canadian TB control directors had to choose one of the regional directors to represent them on the Review Board. Year after year they elected Earl, even though Manitoba was receiving less than five percent of Canada's immigrants for all those years.

Jay Keystone resigned from the Review Board in the mid-1990s because he felt "the government wasn't listening to anything we were saying – they used us as a rubber stamp when they wanted us to say something, and if they didn't, they just ignored us."

By the 1990s, the Review Board was made part of the Department of Justice. Members of the Review Board had to have maximum federal security clearances. Within a short time, though, the Review Board was returned to Citizenship and Immigration Canada. At this point the Justice Department started to set term limits for members of all government committees. Among the longest-serving members, Earl drew the short straw for a position that would turn over first, and so his tenure ended in 2001. He'd been on the Review Board for 23 years, but fighting for immigrants had not worn him out.

EXPORTING KNOWLEDGE

Starting around 1980, when Earl was already involved with national TB programs in southeast Asia, he also got involved with a number of international organizations who worked with immigrants. One of these groups was the Geneva-based International Organization for Migration (IOM). Dr. Brian Gushulak, who was later IOM's medical director, says that Earl reviewed several TB control programs run by IOM in southeast Asia in the late 1980s and early '90s. IOM had one of the largest TB control programs in South Vietnam, dealing with refugee movements after the Vietnam War. Gushulak comments that Earl took the "knowledge he learned in Manitoba and applied it internationally," in this case with his support for IOM.

In 1999, when Gushulak was IOM's Medical Director, Earl was able to demonstrate his support for the organization in a very concrete way. IOM was working on getting the Kosovo refugees out of Macedonia, and to do this they needed pre-departure medical screenings done for thousands of people. Part of the medical screening was for TB, and the local hospitals were swamped, so IOM needed a portable x-ray machine to get the screenings done quickly. IOM didn't have one, and so Gushulak started calling every organization he knew that might have a portable x-ray machine. He called the Union and the World Health Organization in Europe, and then he started calling all over the world. After spending hours on the phone, he thought of Earl in Winnipeg.

Earl's response was immediate. The Manitoba Lung Association had an extra portable x-ray machine that they used to ship up north in a Twin Otter airplane. Earl would not only supply IOM with the x-ray machine, he'd also send his most experienced x-ray technician, Al Harmacy, along to operate it. Al and the portable x-ray machine did "amazing work" in Skopje, Macedonia, and helped ease the refugee crisis there. Gushulak says "those were the kinds of things you never had to worry about asking Earl for."

Another organization Earl became aware of through his work in Asia was the Mennonite Central Committee (MCC). Earl says they "did fantastic work there, without being political; I admired them and learned a lot from them about how to deal with the issues of underprivileged people." Earl wrote a glowing assessment of the MCC's work in Malaysia, where they took refugees already accepted by Canada, looked after their health, taught them English, and helped them learn about Canadian culture. Since MCC's Canadian national office is in Winnipeg, it was a natural step for Earl to begin working with them as an advisor on health issues, which he did through the mid 1980s. Earl met with their Director a number of times a month, and each time they would review six or seven cases. Often Earl would look at x-rays and lab results, and then he would be quoted as an expert advisor in MCC correspondence on behalf of the refugees. Mennonite churches in Manitoba were responsible for sponsoring many Vietnamese refugees to Canada at this time. Earl says that the camps MCC ran in Vietnam were very well-organized and ran excellent directly observed therapy programs for TB: "patients got their treatment and everybody was cured."

The third organization that Earl became aware of on his trips to southeast Asia was Médecins sans Frontières, or Doctors without Borders, who he says were "a wonderful group of people." In the 1980s, this organization was small, mostly French, and mostly concentrated in southeast Asia. Now of course they have expanded all over the world and get mentioned in prime time TV shows like ER.

MORE ADVENTURES ON THE ROAD

In 1988 Earl went to Haiti to evaluate a project funded by Canadian International Development Agency (CIDA). The project was a TB program run by International Child Care, which operated a children's hospital for TB in Port au Prince, and also a TB program in Gonaives. When Earl arrived in Port au Prince, the capital, it was very hot, and every morning he'd take a walk and see one or two dead bodies lying on the main street, covered with tarps. They'd be dragged away for burial, and then it would happen again. By the second week there were four or five bodies on the street each morning, and people started to warn foreigners that the political situation was on the verge of exploding. At midnight on Friday of that week Earl got a telephone call from the Canadian embassy in Port au Prince, advising Earl not to leave the capital, as he'd planned to, because "things are happening." Earl's instructions were to sit tight and not leave the hotel.

Here's what happened later Friday night:

> I was awakened by gunfire and shelling. I didn't know what it was. That afternoon the taxis disappeared from the front of the hotel. This was up in the hills, away from downtown. So at one in the morning I woke up and, stupidly, walked out on the balcony and there about a 1,000 metres away was the presidential palace lit up with gunfire and explosions. I could see tanks. I thought 'what am I standing here for, I might get shot.' I got under the bed and then thought 'what good is that going to do?' So I got dressed and went downstairs and the rest of the guests were

down there too, milling around. The TV in the lobby went off and suddenly the picture of a general came on. Then they played martial music for the next 24 hours.

The general on the TV set was Prosper Avril, who deposed the equally brutal General Henri Namphy. For the next six days, Earl and the other foreigners in the hotel, mostly European businessmen, were trapped. They could see the airport from their windows, and suddenly no planes landed or flew out. The hotel was pleasant, with ample food and drink, but a siege mentality quickly swept through the corridors. Earl says "if I started a rumour it came back to me in one hour, completely different." There were stories that the airport would open immediately, and then that all the white people would be killed. Earl says he wasn't scared, but "I felt a weight on my shoulders." For the last few days of his stay, Earl was able to go back and forth to the International Child Care office in Port au Prince to do his work, and then he flew home to Winnipeg.

Earl had similar luck in the fall of 1982, when he went to a Union meeting in Buenos Aires, Argentina, three months after the Falklands war ended. Earl says that he noticed a lot of noise and a big street demonstration on the plaza, but didn't know why. It turned out to be a march by the mothers of the "disappeared," people who'd been kidnapped and killed by the right-wing military government. This march took place every Wednesday. Earl approached the plaza with a couple of American friends, and the noise kept getting louder. There were armed soldiers and policemen all over the place. Then some soldiers shouted at them to stop, and they pushed all of them against the wall. Earl stuck his hand into his pocket to remove his Canadian passport, "and boy, did they start yelling." They looked at the passport and let Earl go. The Americans didn't have their passports along and they were detained and questioned for a few hours before they got back to the hotel.

Earl was in Peru working on setting up a TB program when violence once again collided with his career, although this time he did finish his work. It was 1997, and Tupac Amaru guerillas kidnapped 400 people attending a reception at the Japanese ambassador's residence in Lima. Luckily for Earl, he wasn't invited.

GUYANA

Currently Earl, who retired from his job as TB Control Director for Manitoba in 2003, is engaged in a large consulting project for the government of Guyana. Assisting him on the project is his long-time Nurse Consultant, Joann MacMorran, also officially retired. The TB work in Guyana is actually part of a larger project that involves sexually transmitted diseases, HIV, and health education. The Canadian Society for International Health approached Earl to act as a consultant on the TB portion.

Earl and Joann went down to Guyana in 2002 to see the situation first-hand. Guyana is poor, a former British colony on the northern edge of South America, and has a large TB problem. The population is about 750,000, highly concentrated in the capital, so it should be possible to create good central control of TB.

Guyana is in the midst of a rampant HIV epidemic, creating a whole population of people co-infected with TB and HIV. Like any region with a lot of latent TB, HIV patients are very likely to get co-infected. There was a TB program already, but it was "piecemeal" and had hardly any laboratory facilities. Medical workers knew how to do smears for microscopic detection of TB, but they had no culture lab. Without such a lab, it's impossible to get a definite diagnosis of TB, or to determine whether there is drug resistance. The Guyanese health care system is so rudimentary that they can't do things North American doctors consider basic, like taking CD4 counts for HIV patients. An additional problem is that there's a transient group of people going back and forth to Britain, the United States and Canada, making contact tracing very difficult.

Earl is directing the establishment of a new TB lab in Guyana, with equipment on order. He and Joann have arranged for residents anywhere in the capital city of Georgetown to get DOTS treatment for TB delivered directly to them. There are 11 DOTS workers, all equipped with mopeds. Normally, no one is hospitalized, so the costs are low. They have set up a training program, made sure there's a drug supply, and set up a training regimen. Drug resistance testing, which requires more sophisticated lab work, will be done in Trinidad and at the National Microbiology Lab in Winnipeg for the foreseeable future.

In addition to working with officials in the Guyanese government and the TB control program, Earl also helped set a teaching curriculum for TB at the university. He and Joann visited chest clinics and saw patients. They met with directors and staff in the TB control program, emphasizing the importance of TB control.

Earl is always curious and well-informed about the places he visits. He observes that the British never had any interest in seeing Guyana develop their economy. Sugar cane was easy to grow and bauxite was easy to mine, but world prices for both commodities have dropped drastically. Agriculture was never developed much, even though pineapple and other fruit could have been grown and processed locally. The British were interested in mining, and Guyana claims that it is developing a "sustainable" mining industry in gold, diamonds and bauxite.

Earl thinks another missed opportunity was setting up a tourist industry. Even though Georgetown's beaches are muddy with river silt, there are beautiful beaches down the coast from the capital. Earl speculates, though, that the dominant political party of the 1990s, the People's Progressive Party, was not interested in tourism.

The People's Progressive Party was run for many years by Cheddi Jaggan, who trained as a dentist in Chicago in the 1940s. In Chicago he met his wife Janet, an American nursing student, and she introduced him to the writings of Marx and

Lenin. In the 1960s, Jaggan was prime minister of the colony of Guiana, with Janet as minister of health. Then from 1964 to 1992, Guyanese elections were rigged by parties funded and encouraged by the Americans, who were desperately scared that the left-wing Jaggan would win.

On Earl's visit in spring 2004, he indulged his interests in politics and people and met Janet Jagan:

> We had a very nice chat. She's Jewish, but a secular Jew. She was president for two years after Cheddi Jagan died in 1997. I asked her why the government didn't develop the tourist industry, but she didn't really answer the question. Very interesting woman though. I had read about her for years.

Thanks to British indifference and American interference, the Guyanese economy has been in shambles for many years and something like a third of the population has left for Canada, the US, Trinidad, and England. Earl, who is a practical doctor and not just a part-time historian, says that "the reason you have to do TB control in Guyana is because we have a lot of Guyanese immigrants in Canada with TB that they were infected with at home. You've got to look at the program in Guyana to stop them from getting infected."

RESEARCH ON THE HOME FRONT

"MOST TB CONTROL OFFICERS ARE NOT ENGAGED IN CLINICAL RESEARCH
AND DON'T HAVE MUCH OF A CLUE ABOUT IT. SOMEONE LIKE EARL
WHO RECOGNIZED THE IMPORTANCE OF RESEARCH IN A PROGRAM SETTING,
IMPROVED THE QUALITY OF THE PROGRAM AND THE SERVICES IT PROVIDES
TO PATIENTS. IF WE COULD HAVE HAD MORE OF EARL'S TYPE CDC WOULD
HAVE BEEN ABLE TO ACCOMPLISH EVEN MORE IN THE LAST FEW YEARS."
— DR. RICK O'BRIEN, FORMER HEAD OF TB RESEARCH
AT THE CENTERS FOR DISEASE CONTROL

Earl's research work spans a four decade period, and one of his interests has always been immigrants and TB. "Earl and other colleagues in the 1980s and during the early part of his career did some of the basic epidemiological work on TB in Canadian immigrants," says Brian Gushulak, Citizenship and Immigration's Medical Director. Since 1988 Earl's biggest research projects have been funded by the Centers for Disease Control (CDC) in Atlanta.

Earl and his research team applied for their first CDC grant in 1988, which was to be the first part of an ongoing relationship. Within two years they became the first Canadian site to participate in CDC's multi-centre studies, which allowed them to access on-going funds from CDC so they could maintain a full-time staff, even between research projects. The Health Sciences Centre in Winnipeg continued to be the only Canadian site for CDC's TB research until 1999. CDC adopted the multi-centre model simply because TB had become too rare in North America to get enough patients "enrolled" as subjects in a study in any one site.

Dr. Wayne Kepron, a lung disease specialist who has worked with Earl for many years, says that Winnipeg became the first Canadian site for this research partly because its population was small enough that the city could have a certain amount of TB but keep it under good control, and also because Winnipeg had a long tradition of keeping really solid TB statistics. Earl was a big part of the reason for those solid statistics.

Earl's projects are part of two CDC research consortia, one the TB Trials Consortium (TBTC), and the other the TB Epidemiological Studies Consortium (TBESC). The TBTC conducts clinical drug trials, and the TBESC consortium does studies on how TB is spread. At this point the TBTC consortium has 22 sites in the US, three in Canada, and single sites in Brazil, Spain, and Uganda. The TBESC sites largely overlap with these. Earl is the principal investigator, or PI in the scientific jargon, for all the Winnipeg projects funded by CDC.

Since 1988, Earl's team has brought in about $10 million in grant money and employs seven professional staff full-time. The University of Manitoba administers the grants. The first project, in 1988, was to study people with latent TB. A second grant, in 1994, went to Earl's group for a trial of the first new TB drug in 25 years, rifapentine. It was approved by the FDA in 1998.

Right now the TB Trials Consortium in Winnipeg is working actively on multiple CDC studies. One of them is in a follow-up phase, tracking patients who took a new treatment regimen for HIV and TB co-infection. Another study is a new, six month, three-drug regimen for patients who are resistant to one of the standard TB drugs or cannot tolerate it. Earl's team is also conducting a study of latent TB in immigrants, which is designed to shorten the treatment regimen to three months for those who do not have active disease. Nine months of taking drugs with serious side effects is a long time for people who feel perfectly well. The idea is to kill the latent TB bugs in one-third the time of current drug treatments. Finally, the team is working on a drug trial using moxifloxacin, a new drug that has the potential to treat active TB in the first two months.

Concurrently, Earl's TBESC group is involved in a number of studies of how TB is spread. One of them looks at risk factors for how TB may spread from patients to their contacts. Another deals with immunogenetic susceptibility to TB, something that can be studied in a truly scientific way now with DNA fingerprinting and other modern laboratory tools. This group will soon be working on a study involving drug-resistant TB as well.

The sheer scope of this research activity is staggering. The staggering became quite literal when Earl's filing cabinets needed to be moved when he retired as TB control director in 2003. I helped move many of the boxes to the basement of the Respiratory Hospital at HSC so that I could carry on with my research for this book. The correspondence, grant applications, enrollment lists, patient files and so on for these projects spilled endlessly out of boxes that were too small for all the paper. Marian Roth, who has been working on Earl's research projects since 1999, says simply that "TB is Dr. Hershfield's life."

9

HOPE

"IT'S CHEAPER TO PREVENT THE FIRE THAN TO PUT IT OUT"
— BONO, U2 SINGER AND ACTIVIST, SPEAKING ABOUT THE AFRICAN AIDS EPIDEMIC
AT THE LIBERAL LEADERSHIP CONVENTION ON NOVEMBER 14, 2003

New risks and an increasing burden of disease are the story of TB today, but they are not the whole story by any means. Most people don't know that millions of people with AIDS are actually killed by TB, and that TB needs to be treated first among the co-infected. Public awareness and the politics of public health are crucial for making change happen with this disease. As Canadians, we need to think about whether we believe that health is a universal human right, and what it means to be global citizens. Any hope we might have for beating TB rests not just with the new medical developments I discuss, but also with the people who deliver health care. In the end, any moral imperative for change will have to come from each one of us.

There are many reasons to be hopeful about the future of tuberculosis control both in Canada and beyond. There are at least as many reasons to be worried. The statistics continue to be grim in the 22 "high-burden" countries that get 80% of the world's TB. When four people die every minute from a single, curable disease, that is reasonable cause for concern. However, two of the problems that experts thought would explode globally in the 1990s have so far stayed largely out of the developed world. Those problems are widespread co-infection of HIV and TB, and a global outbreak of multi-drug-resistant TB. Those of us living in North America and Europe may well find ourselves dodging an increasing hail of bullets on both those issues. Immigration, international travel and trade, vicious regional wars, increasing poverty, and over-strained public health systems all put us at risk for a global TB epidemic.

Dr. Arnold Naimark, former dean of the University of Manitoba's medical school, sees the history of TB control as divisible into two main eras. The first one started in the late 19th century and ended around 1950, and actually saw the most rapid decline in TB rates ever recorded. The reductions were likely achieved by better nutrition, improved health care, and less crowded housing. The second era began in 1950 with the introduction of effective antibiotics to treat the disease, which caused a second but less dramatic decline. Public perception shifted accordingly:

> Tuberculosis was in the minds of people as a major killer, often of young people, and literature is full of young people dying of tuberculosis as one of the tragic events in novels, plays and later in film. It was very much in the public mind just the way that diphtheria and scarlet fever were. That has changed completely. Hardly anyone you can talk to knows anybody who has TB – except in certain socioeconomic groups. Where it would have been common for someone in the family to have had active TB, now it's quite rare, and has become in the last couple of decades a disease that people only think of in relation to special populations, either Aboriginals or refugees from Vietnam and the far east and so forth. So it's seen as 'somebody else's disease' and not one in the predominantly white population. That's been a huge change in consciousness.

Naimark thinks people should know two things about TB. First, they should understand a little about the history of the disease and the resurgence of TB in the 1980s and '90s, when it has once again predominantly affected younger people in their most productive years. Second, they should know that TB is a disease with "a much higher incidence in other parts of the world, where, as world citizens, we need to be concerned about international health and stability, because in the long run we pay for it if it isn't controlled."

The geography of TB is going to make control difficult. Because the disease is especially prevalent in countries that are poor and even suffering some sort of collapse, whether due to war, environmental issues, or just poverty, it is inevitable that people will flee those countries carrying the disease. These refugees will seek a better life, as so many Canadians have over the last century, in a richer country. They will bring their TB with them.

NEW RISKS WITH AN OLD DISEASE

The AIDS epidemic is amplifying the world's current TB epidemic. TB numbers are going up 10% a year where they would likely only increase 3% a year without the presence of HIV infection. The World Health Organization's most current estimates of people co-infected with the deadly combination of HIV and TB is 11 million, but the significance of this is lost on many AIDS activists. For example, Bono, front man for rock group U2, has become an impassioned and effective advocate for the cause of African AIDS sufferers. However, if you search the "Debt, AIDS, Trade, Africa" web site[7] for the word "tuberculosis," you will find only a few passing references in the archives section. Yet 68% of people co-infected globally are African, and those who develop TB and AIDS will die, on average, within five weeks. In Africa, Asia and South America at least a third of deaths attributed to AIDS are actually caused by TB, and even international health organizations waste time fighting about the statistics. Yet the deadly synergy between these diseases points clearly to the fact that you cannot fight AIDS in areas with high TB incidence without also fighting TB.

Once TB is endemic in a population, it lurks, waiting for the best chance to strike. Infectious disease doctors talk about TB as an "AIDS-defining illness" because when someone has active TB it often points to the presence of AIDS – the TB has just seized on its best opportunity, which is a broken immune system. Anne Fanning of the University of Alberta's school of medicine explains how latent TB infection works when you have an AIDS epidemic. TB latency, she says, makes you think you have the disease controlled, and any re-emergence would be on a case-by-case basis "unless there were some other disease – like AIDS – that enables an entire population of previously infected people to re-activate. That's what's happening in Africa."

Dr. Frank Plummer, director of Winnipeg's Centre for Infectious Disease Prevention and Control, spent 17 years in Kenya doing research on HIV. He says that

> the epidemic of HIV and the epidemic of tuberculosis feed off each other. If you have HIV you're more likely to reactivate TB infection and more likely to acquire a new TB infection. In a community with co-infection, people who don't have HIV also become more likely to get TB.

I asked him if he thinks progress is being made against HIV in Africa, and he said "the epidemic shows no signs of abating, and it's also spreading into new areas, like India and China, at alarming rates."

Dr. Lee Jong-Wook, the head of the World Health Organization, was quoted in an Associated Press story in late April 2004 saying "it's difficult to grasp the magnitude of the [AIDS] problem. The 8,000 people dying every day from AIDS is equivalent to 30 jumbo jets crashing every day." He also warned against seeing the AIDS epidemic as only an African problem, citing growing case numbers in Eastern Europe, Russia, southeast Asia, Thailand, Vietnam, Indonesia and Singapore. What he did not say was that these all happen to be countries with high incidence of tuberculosis.

---

[7] The Debt, AIDS, Trade, Africa web site can be found at <www.data.org>.

The other new risk on the horizon for TB control is multi-drug-resistant (MDR) TB, which the World Health Organization estimates that 50 million people are infected with worldwide. As with co-infection, those of us in the developed world can easily be oblivious to this problem since it is so rare here. In Canada, there are only 15-20 cases per year, but this is the tip of a global iceberg. Russia produces large amounts of multi-drug-resistant TB in their massive, overcrowded prison system, and nobody has any idea how much of it gets exported. The deadly irony with MDR is that treating and beating it requires the most resources, the newest drugs, and the most sophisticated lab work. Exactly the things that are lacking in the places it most commonly occurs.

CO-INFECTION AT HOME

Ann Russell is an outpatient nurse at Winnipeg's Health Sciences Centre, where she has worked with HIV patients since 1990. She also works with the still-rare patients who are co-infected with TB. Patients are referred by family physicians, walk-in clinics, or by other parts of the hospital. Ann is the front-line contact for patients, and she collaborates with infectious disease doctors to make sure that patients get the right treatment.

Anyone who is co-infected with HIV and TB has to take a lot of pills. Co-infected patients take drugs three times a day, with regimens up to 18 pills a day. The hospital can't afford to provide directly observed therapy (DOT) for these patients, so instead pharmacies bubble-pack medications and hospital staff check their used bubble-packs to make sure all the pills are gone. Obviously this doesn't guarantee compliance the way DOT does, but success rates have been good.

Success rates have been high with co-infected patients for a number of reasons. First, Ann ensures that the patient is ready to make a commitment to their treatment, as well as finding out if there are substance abuse issues that might interfere with patients coming in for treatment. Therapy does not begin immediately after diagnosis, which was the practice in the 1990s. Second, the two diseases have to be dealt with in the right order: co-infected patients get their TB treated first, since TB is the more infectious of the two diseases and because the TB needs to be under control before HIV therapy can work properly. In addition, HIV and TB drugs have the potential for very nasty interactions, so it's best not to overlap HIV treatment with the most intense part of the TB drug regimen in the first two months.

Ann sees what she believes to be disproportionate numbers of Aboriginal people diagnosed with HIV, and of course they are also at increased risk for TB. Sometimes she sees clusters of co-infected patients who have likely infected each other. These include Aboriginal people and the homeless.

The people most at risk for getting HIV, Ann feels, are the least likely to understand how to prevent it. She observes that HIV is "a stigmatizing disease" for many immigrants, who are "terrified of being ostracized by other members of their community." Ann says "there are a lot of closed doors to people who really need to understand how transmission of HIV works." If patients have trouble understanding HIV transmission, co-infection with TB represents a terrifying escalation of complexity and stigmatization. And the numbers are going up in Canada too.

WHAT YOU SHOULD KNOW

Many of the doctors and international health experts I spoke to when writing this book said different versions of the same thing: TB is not glamorous and only gets attention when there's a flare-up in the developed world. The dreaded U-shaped curve that infectious disease doctors talk about plots incidence of disease against time, and what it demonstrates is really a social phenomenon more than a medical one. As a disease like TB appears to be under control, with rates dropping on the left-hand side of the U-shaped curve, the public and even public health authorities stop paying attention. By taking their eyes off the ball, they help create the conditions for the resurgence of the disease, the right-hand side of the U-shaped curve, which inevitably becomes harder to treat than the last round was.

TB control experts are a bit like a fire department that only fights fires that are invisible to most taxpayers. No one hears the sirens or sees the flames. Kevin Elwood, director of TB control in British Columbia, said

> the people who get TB largely don't have any kind of lobby, except for the HIV community in cases of co-infection. At the same time with the limited number of cases there's no reason the public should have a large awareness of TB unless it directly affects them.

Anne Fanning, of the University of Alberta's medical school, explains how public health departments need to remain vigilant even though the public has lost awareness of a disease. She used the example of Ontario closing chest clinics and reducing capacity to deal with TB in the 1980s. By the late 1990s they were rebuilding their program in downtown Toronto. Fanning believes that there has to be "a way to maintain expertise" when a disease is under control. She said "we have to create surge capacity. It's an interesting concept in public health but it applies in the SARS situation, with the avian flu, and with TB."

Lee Reichman, who runs the New Jersey Medical School National TB Center, is probably the most articulate and impassioned advocate for tuberculosis care in the world. Here's what he said when I asked him what the public should know about TB:

> They should know that it's the biggest single killer of any infection worldwide, and the paradox is that it's always been so, and it's totally preventable and curable. TB has got an image problem – it's extremely

under-appreciated. TB kills two million a year, and that's just because the WHO needed some people to die from AIDS, so they took 2 million people from the TB column and put them in AIDS. You compare that to when people get excited about SARS, which in 2003 killed 813, the Ebola epidemic of about five years ago that killed 245, West Nile in the United States that killed 232, and anthrax that killed five. Yet those are the kinds of things we get excited about, but we don't get excited about TB. It's because it's a disease of the poor, of the developing world, but people should realize that just because it's over there doesn't mean it couldn't affect us over here.

As Reichman points out, the TB that people keep forgetting about is mostly abroad, and it keeps coming to the developed world with immigrants and refugees. How will we control a disease that increasingly originates beyond our borders? Dr. Frank Plummer, whose Winnipeg disease centre works on the whole range of infectious diseases, makes this argument for Canada's involvement in what might appear to be other people's problems:

SARS pointed out very vividly that the front lines of infectious disease control may well be overseas. So having an active role in many infectious diseases that are threats primarily elsewhere is an important thing for this country in terms of its own health security. We can't rely on others to do it.

I think that Canada as part of the global community has an obligation to contribute to global health efforts, partly out of enlightened self-interest, and partly because it's our responsibility as global citizens.

IS HEALTH A HUMAN RIGHT?

In what appears to be a bizarre irony, the same World Bank that in 1993 endorsed DOT, or directly observed therapy, as a cost-effective virtual vaccine-substitute for treating TB, also thinks that patients in the world's poorest countries should pay for their DOT treatment. The irony is that one of the principles of DOT from the beginning has been that it is free; there are arm-loads of research that shows patients abandoning their treatment when they have to pay. If you read this research literature, you might not even notice its authors are angry about this issue, but they are. Here's what Rick O'Brien, former head of TB research at CDC says about "cost recovery" (i.e. making patients pay for treatment):

cost recovery in the health sector is being promoted in lower income countries as part of economic reforms required by external lending institutions such as the World Bank and the International Monetary Fund.

The costs the lenders are not interested in are the ones that are harder to quantify. What does it cost a society if it does not make health a human right? Maybe the lenders should just start counting the cost of all that lost productivity, if the rhetoric of human rights is uncomfortable for them. They could also try counting the money actually collected from poor people for "cost recovery in the health sector." The chances are it will drive away people who need treatment without recovering program costs. That's not a good medical or financial formula.

In the United States, the medical system is industrialized and wants a lot more than cost recovery — they want profits. Lee Reichman comments simply that "you can't make money from public health." He thinks it would be very difficult to make a profit from contact investigation for TB, but that doesn't mean public health systems should stop doing it. When I asked him whether he thinks the American system of private insurance is a good way of controlling infectious diseases, he said "private medical care is incompatible with public health."

Other American health care experts like Bess Miller and Sara Rosenbaum have expressed similar skepticism about the ability of the private, "managed care" system to effectively control TB in particular. When it comes to outbreak and contact investigations, for example, managed care organizations are more worried about your insurance status than your health status. As people change jobs or move or become unemployed, their file moves to different managed care companies, or they lose their insurance. Why would a managed care organization bother investigating TB contacts who are not enrolled with their organization? After all, managed care companies are responsible only to their shareholders. It used to be that public health had as its shareholders everyone who lived in the society. If that's not true anymore, Americans will need to understand the consequences for infectious disease control.

Everyone agrees that the world needs new TB drugs, but the tough question is: who pays the bill? Opinions differ on the obligations of big pharmaceutical companies to provide new TB drugs at low cost. Rick O'Brien says "it's easy to blame the drug companies, but they have to answer to their stockholders." He goes on to laud Aventis South Africa for its grant to the Medical Research Council, and Eli Lilly for slashing the price of some second-line TB drugs by 95%. He also mentions Bayer, which is collaborating with CDC in a new drug trial. Paul Farmer, a doctor who helped lobby Eli Lilly into reducing some of its TB drug prices, is less impressed with big pharma's obligations to its stockholders. He cites a 2001 report that found "all of the nine US pharmaceutical companies that market the top-selling 50 drugs for seniors spent more money on marketing, advertising, and administration than they did on R&D."

OH CANADA

Canadians like to complain about their health care system, and sometimes look enviously to the south, where people get tests and procedures with the latest equipment really fast – as long as they can pay for it and their HMO allows it. But the United States currently spends almost 15% of its GDP on health care while leaving 40 million of its citizens without health insurance. Canada spends 10% of GDP on health care and insures 100% of its citizens through publicly-funded medicare. Maybe we're not doing so badly.

Dr. Gordon Guyatt, a professor in the faculty of health sciences at McMaster University, noted in a recent *Globe and Mail* editorial that if lowering taxes trumps all other considerations, then we indeed have a problem with medicare. With this ideology, spending more on health care while receiving less for our money won't matter. Private pay is the only solution if lower taxes are a higher priority than public health. But what about the much-discussed innovation of privately delivered health care that is still publicly funded? When I asked Guyatt about that idea, he told me that

> It would be a big mistake. The evidence clearly shows when you compare private for-profit and private not-for-profit hospitals in the United States there are increased death rates in for-profit hospitals, the reason being that they need 15% of their money to generate a profit, as well as higher payments to executives and CEOs. The result is that they have to skimp on services, and what our work summarizing the literature showed is that in both hospital settings and outpatient dialysis settings, the result of that skimping is higher death rates for patients.

Ontario has of course experimented with lowering taxes and slashing healthcare budgets during the 1990s. Earl and other TB doctors told me about how decentralizing the TB program there reduced its effectiveness. Judge Archie Campbell's report on Ontario's recent SARS crisis has language that might chasten those who are eager to put the squeeze on our healthcare system:

> SARS showed Ontario's central public-health system to be unprepared, fragmented, poorly led, uncoordinated, inadequately resourced, professionally impoverished, and generally incapable of discharging its mandate.

WILL WE EVER BEAT IT?

"When I read material about elimination of TB it gives me
the heeby jeebies because the rates are still going up globally
and if we neglect it globally we can't possibly hope for elimination,
so it's that kind of talk I think neglects the rest of the world."
— Anne Fanning

"Tuberculosis will persist; people will forget.
Do we want this to be our legacy?"
— Rick O'Brien, "Tuberculosis in the Future"

TB is a disease that lulls those of us in the developed world to sleep with a seductive U-curve, tempting politicians and public health officials to ignore it. The irony is that we only talk about eliminating TB when there's a resurgence of the disease in rich countries. TB was killing people in developing countries throughout the 20th century in huge numbers. But with global numbers going steadily downwards in the 1970s, people overlooked mortality figures that were still disturbing and confidently predicted eventual elimination of the disease. By the mid-1980s, the World Health Organization's TB program in Geneva had only two staff members: one statistician to count the deaths and one secretary to write them down. Then in 1989, the Centers for Disease Control in the United States made a dramatic declaration of the elimination of TB in the US, and almost immediately the American rates started going up. All of a sudden TB was in the headlines of New York newspapers and on the cover of *Newsweek*. What distressed North Americans about this trend was that members of the middle class were getting the disease – prison guards, health care workers, teachers, commuters on subways. All of a sudden politicians were willing to spend money on TB control after a decade or more of de-funding programs.

Complacency in politicians and the public is understandable. But in our complacency, we all expect public health programs to remain vigilant on our behalf. The problem is that when disease rates are low, public health still needs money and resources from complacent politicians and taxpayers. And it can happen again. Philip Hopewell of the University of California explains it like this:

It's going to get increasingly difficult to argue for support for TB control as the case rate gets lower. Yet it requires continued attention. The resurgence in the late 1980s and early '90s demonstrated that very clearly. Take your eye off the ball and it hits you in the head.

Frank Plummer says that "we've seen time and again that once you stop investing, infectious diseases come back."

I asked various TB doctors and experts if they thought tuberculosis would ever be eliminated globally. Earl Hershfield doesn't think so. George Comstock, the Johns Hopkins epidemiologist, said "maybe a couple thousand years from now. I wouldn't be surprised to see a repeat of the 1990s in the US and perhaps in other developed countries too." Comstock and Frank Plummer talked about political will. It was the same mantra Earl learned doing international work: if the national government was unwilling to commit resources to the program, you couldn't control TB.

Another reason for the curse of the U-shaped curve is that doctors in low-incidence countries have trouble diagnosing the disease, because they see it so rarely. I talked to a nurse who said she worked with patients who went to the doctor three or four times and got treated for pneumonia before their TB was finally recognized. Kevin Elwood in BC says "you can be a family physician in this province and go for years without seeing a case… the presentation can be rather non-specific, a cough for six weeks, a flu. How do you separate the coughs from the one that happens to be TB?"

On the global stage the World Health Organization has set targets of detecting 70% of new infectious TB cases and curing 85% of detected cases by 2005. However, in 2002 only 44% of the estimated number of TB patients were getting detected world-wide. The patients who got directly observed therapy, or DOTS, had a cure rate of 82%, almost at the target. But the only country in the world with a high burden of TB that has met the World Health Organization targets is Vietnam. The African region has a treatment success rate of only 71% of detected cases, largely because of AIDS co-infection. And no one knows exactly how many undetected cases there are in Africa. In Eastern Europe treatment success for detected cases of TB is only 70%, in their case because of drug resistance issues.

HOPE FOR THE FUTURE

"WE HAVE A REMARKABLY REWARDING DISEASE TO TREAT. WE CURE PEOPLE!
WHEREAS THE ASTHMAS AND THE OBSTRUCTIVE LUNG DISEASE
AND THE LUNG CANCERS AND ALL OF THAT, YOU DON'T. YOUNG COLLEAGUES
OFTEN WANT TO DO GLAMOROUS THINGS, BUT THEY DON'T REALIZE
THAT THE TREATMENT OF TUBERCULOSIS IS VERY REWARDING."
— KEVIN ELWOOD, DIRECTOR OF TB CONTROL IN BRITISH COLUMBIA

There are many reasons to be hopeful about getting TB under control, in spite of the depressing reality of global mortality and infection statistics. More money than ever before is going into TB research and control. There are also exciting initiatives to find new and better TB drugs, vaccines, and diagnostics. Any hope for these initiatives must be tempered with the realization that an enormous and unwavering effort will be needed.

In retrospect, 1998's sequencing of the complete genome of *mycobacterium tuberculosis* may seem as significant as Robert Koch's discovery of the TB bacillus in 1882. The reason we will need hindsight to assess the significance of this discovery, though, is because everything depends on what's done with this new information. Development of new drugs, a new vaccine, and new diagnostic tools should all be aided by the sequencing of the TB genome. Earl and all the TB experts I spoke to believe that TB can only be brought under control with large advances in these areas.

New drugs are needed to shorten the course of treatment, which currently stands at six-nine months. This is still a long time to take medications, even if there were no side effects. Another goal of new drugs is to reduce the time patients are contagious with TB. Finally, new drugs are needed because there is too much resistance to the old ones already out there. When it appeared in 1998, rifapentine was the first new TB drug to come out in over 20 years. But there may be others soon. Better, shorter therapies for treatment of latent TB infection are also needed to replace the current ones.

As for a new vaccine, Earl says "I hope it's like the smallpox vaccine — take it once and that's it." That is certainly not the case with BCG vaccine today. Many of the doctors I spoke to believe an effective vaccine is only a decade away. If that's true, Earl believes control programs can then "concentrate all our efforts on giving preventive therapy to infected people." A new vaccine is also widely believed to be the best possible approach to preventing multi-drug-resistant strains of TB.

Computer modeling studies show that even a vaccine that is 50-70% efficacious would, combined with drug therapy, save tens of millions of lives. BCG vaccine, which has been around since 1921, is nowhere near that effective. Given the fact that many people are infected with TB but have a normal immune response that protects them from getting sick with the disease, it should be possible to mimic that natural immune response with a vaccine. Several new vaccine candidates for TB have been developed in recent years and shown promising results with animal testing.

The Aeras Global TB Vaccine Foundation in Maryland is the only organization dedicated to producing a new TB vaccine. Their goal is to have a new TB vaccine on the world market within 10 years and they are well on the way. Already they have manufactured and performed the pre-clinical evaluation and regulatory activities for a new recombinant BCG vaccine candidate for first phase trials. Aeras has established clinical research sites in Cape Town, South Africa, the United States, and Europe, where they will test candidate vaccines.

In terms of new diagnostic tools, one of the problems has always been to distinguish TB infection from the trace infection caused by BCG vaccination. One new product now being investigated is quantiferon, which has an immunological marker that you can measure, giving a clear reading of whether someone has TB infection. It even has the potential to predict who will go on to get active TB once they're infected.

Rick O'Brien, who's now scientific director for the Foundation for Innovative New Diagnostics, or FIND, in Geneva, summed up what's needed to get TB under control:

> We still need more resources, just to beef up programs. We need more technical expertise. And most importantly and fundamentally we need new tools. Just the fact that TB therapy hasn't changed much in twenty odd years, that we're relying on a diagnostic test, smear microscopy, that's been around for a hundred years, and the vaccine that's available doesn't work very well, is pretty good proof that we badly need new tools and continued research.

O'Brien believes that better TB diagnostics are a major priority. His organization wants to get a new diagnostic test for TB done in a relatively short time that could also be a model for other infectious diseases like malaria and possibly HIV. Like a number of the new health research organizations, FIND is partnering with private sector companies.

"The focus," says O'Brien, "is on more rapid and accurate tests for the diagnosis of active TB." They are also interested in finding "more rapid ways of assessing drug resistance, particularly rifampin resistance, that usually equates with multi-drug-resistant TB." He describes FIND as having "a social mission but employing capitalistic business practices in advancing that mission."

Bill Gates, most famous as the billionaire owner of Microsoft, has become a big name in disease research through his foundation. The Bill & Melinda Gates Foundation has awarded tens of millions of dollars to TB and AIDS research, including support for O'Brien's FIND organization and for research the University of Manitoba is doing on AIDS in Africa. The Gates Foundation has also provided the Aeras organization with a grant of $82.9 million US for new TB vaccine development.

Then there is the Geneva-based Global Fund to Fight AIDS, Tuberculosis, and Malaria. The Global Fund is a funding mechanism rather than a program or research organization. Currently they are supporting a huge scale-up of HIV treatment, including a six-fold increase in Africa. The Global Fund is also funding treatment for drug-resistant malaria, and helping rebuild the war-shattered TB program in Sierra Leone. Canada has contributed $100 million US to this initiative originally begun at a G-8 summit.

Another new organization is the Global Alliance for Tuberculosis Drug Development, headquartered in New York. As their name implies, they are focused on developing new TB drugs. The idea for the alliance started in 2000, at a conference to promote the development of new TB drugs held in Cape Town, South Africa. The conference brought together TB experts, pharmaceutical companies, the World Health Organization, and funders. Lee Reichman, never content to just complain from the sidelines, was involved from the beginning and is now on the board of directors, as is Rick O'Brien. The Gates Foundation has again come through, this time with more than $40 million.

The Cape Town meeting recognized something very important about the future of TB, which was that DOTS alone would not beat the disease — new drugs are also needed. Directly observed therapy evolved largely to ensure the effectiveness of drugs that were far from perfect. There remains an extraordinary problem with the length and complexity of TB treatment, and now that many of the same patients also have to be treated for AIDS, things are even worse.

The Global Alliance has three goals in terms of new drug development for TB. First and most important, new drugs need to be found that will allow shortened and simplified therapy. Second, new drugs are needed to treat multi-drug-resistant TB. Last, they want to treat latent TB infection better than is done now; this is mostly an issue in developed countries.

Dr. Maria C. Freire, chief executive officer of the Global Alliance, says that "for 40 years, TB drug development was at standstill. Today, we have a robust pipeline which is a quantum leap from where the world was three years ago." Like FIND and Aeras, they are able to move quickly because they are a non-profit organization dedicated to a single focus.

PA824 is the new TB drug the Global Alliance has farthest along in development. PA824 was originally developed by another company and used in cancer research in India. The Global Alliance licensed the drug from the company that owned it for a relatively nominal amount of money, and that company retains the right to co-develop the drug if there is a good financial opportunity to do that. They expect to begin clinical trails for PA824 in 2005 in South Africa. Currently the Global Alliance has ten anti-TB compounds in their portfolio, and they want to double that.

Even with all this new money and technology being deployed on TB, controlling the disease will not get done without human resources. We need experienced people to build TB control programs all over the world, people who have careers like Earl Hershfield's. Philip Hopewell, who has also worked internationally on TB programs, is primarily concerned that developing countries get the technical assistance they need to organize effective programs:

> My concern at an international level is that at least right now there's a lot of money going into TB control without adequate technical assistance and oversight. We've continually complained about insufficient attention and insufficient funding and now with the Global Fund and various other initiatives there's a lot of money. I'm concerned that things won't be done right otherwise.

Talking to someone like Hopewell, who has worked on TB control for many years, is sobering. You can spend hours looking at the splashy, colourful web sites for all the ambitious, well-funded TB programs, and forget the facts on the ground: millions of people dying every year from a living, ancient, curable and preventable disease. The fact that we rarely see the victims of TB makes them easy to forget, but disease crosses borders and gates. Not just corporations become global forces.

Tuberculosis is not somebody else's problem. But until those of us who live in the world's wealthiest countries take ownership of this problem, there is no hope that tuberculosis will stop killing millions of people all over the world, including some right here at home.

AFTERWORD

I f the hiring of Earl Hershfield in 1967 was a watershed for the history of TB control in Manitoba, then his retirement as director of the program at the end of 2003 may represent a similar opportunity. There may never again be changes in Manitoba's TB program as momentous as the universal implementation of drug treatment, or the closing of the Ninette sanatorium, but there are other significant changes converging in 2005. One of them is the ongoing resurgence of the disease among Aboriginal people in the province, especially in northern communities. Another is the small but disturbing number of people co-infected with HIV and TB. Finally the issues in various immigrant communities with TB continue in Manitoba, but the cultural complexity of dealing with the medical problem is increasing as we see immigrants coming from different places than they did in the 1970s and '80s. A tiny percentage of these immigrants bring drug-resistant strains of TB with them, and occasionally they are co-infected with HIV. At the same time, the establishment of the Centre for Infectious Disease Prevention and Control in Winnipeg should lead to new opportunities for Manitoba to be a leader in TB control. How will the Manitoba TB control program respond to these challenges and opportunities?

I visited the new director of TB control for Manitoba, Dr. Pam Orr, in her office at the Health Sciences Centre in Winnipeg shortly after she started in the position. I wanted to ask Orr about how she would handle the immediate challenges of TB control, especially in the Manitoba populations with high disease rates – Aboriginal and immigrant communities.

I asked Orr first about her approach to TB control. She talked about sharing data and experience with the other western provinces: "we share with Alberta and Saskatchewan our situation in terms of Aboriginal communities and difficulty in terms of remote communities." Orr herself has worked in First Nations communities as a physician, and she has done research work in Brazil, Burma, and Laos on sexually transmitted diseases.

In working with the Aboriginal community, Orr wants to emphasize "creating a partnership with the person who's ill," rather than simply telling people what to do. She feels there is "lingering anger and disappointment" in the Aboriginal community about the paternalistic approach taken by health officials in the past. She recognizes, however, that it is difficult to balance the public health aspect of TB with a less authoritarian approach:

> Chasing people around an Aboriginal community or Winnipeg's core area and telling them that if they don't show up to take their pills they'll be apprehended is sometimes a situation we have to envisage. It doesn't really help in terms of creating a trusting relationship. In the First Nations communities in the north and in the core area, I don't have a magic solution for that other than continuing to try to have a respectful conversation.

One change she has implemented already is that some TB patients from northern communities are being treated at their home nursing station. Orr wants to build expertise in district hospitals like Thompson and Churchill so patients don't always have to spend months in Winnipeg for their initial treatment phase.

When it comes to working with immigrants who have TB, Orr believes there is "still a knowledge and trust gap between immigrants and program workers." The problem begins, says Orr, when recent immigrants who tested positive for TB infection on arrival get a notice from the provincial health department telling them to report to a Winnipeg clinic. At the clinic "they're somewhat confused and a bit scared." She thinks this anxiety could be defused by working with immigrant groups so people in the community would know more about the disease and the public health measures used to control it. Orr also believes this kind of education might get people who have active disease to report to the clinic earlier. She wants to work with refugee organizations and doctors who are in minority communities to disseminate information about TB and the process of tracking and treating it.

I asked Orr about how concerned she was with co-infection of HIV and TB in Manitoba. She said she is very concerned, not because the numbers are high, but because of how hard it is to treat those individuals who are likely to be co-infected:

> These individuals are hard to find for contact tracing, and hard to do skin-testing on. Then they're very hard to treat. They've tuned out of the regular world and values. They're poor and involved in crime or the sex trade. Some of them are from minority groups. In this time when social services is burdened with an increasing load, it's hard to reach these individuals. There aren't resources to reach this group. We're seeing an increasing group of disenfranchised individuals.

There's a gentleman in the ward upstairs who says that he does not want to stop his crystal methamphetamine habit, but he will take his TB medicines. So of course we know when he gets out and gets high on crystal meth, he won't come for his TB treatment. He'll forget. So what do you do with these people? Lock them up?

Orr sees this as "a challenge to the limits of freedom in society," but not a new dilemma. She believes the American public health system has consistently been more authoritarian when faced with this kind of problem.

At the end of the interview, Orr says that she's optimistic about the future of the program, and what an honour it is to work with the staff she inherited from Earl Hershfield. Orr stands up in her white lab coat and shakes my hand forcefully. She answers the telephone as I leave the office. There are x-rays to read.

BIBLIOGRAPHIC NOTES

The best introductory book for the general reader about tuberculosis is *Timebomb: The Global Epidemic of Multi-Drug-Resistant Tuberculosis,* by Lcc Reichman with Janice Hopkins Tanne (McGraw-Hill, 2002). Reichman conveys the urgency of the contemporary problem with the disease while also doing a superb job of explaining the history and science of TB. I also recommend the vividly written chapter on tuberculosis in Andrew Nikiforuk's book, *The Fourth Horseman: A short history of plagues, scourges and emerging viruses* (Penguin, 1991). For more in-depth coverage on the whole gamut of topics related to TB control, there is *Tuberculosis: A Comprehensive International Approach,* edited by Lee Reichman and Earl Hershfield (Marcel Dekker, 2nd edition, 2000). It is the definitive textbook on TB control, but readable as well for those of us without medical training. There are many general books on the history of TB. One that I drew on was Thomas M. Daniel's *Captain of Death: The Story of Tuberculosis* (University of Rochester Press, 1997).

No one could write about TB in Canada without reading George Jasper Wherrett's *The Miracle of the Empty Beds: A History of Tuberculosis in Canada* (University of Toronto Press, 1977). Wherrett's Royal Commission study, *Tuberculosis in Canada,* was also a valuable reference for me (Queen's Printer, 1965). For a modern, sociologically-oriented view, Katherine McCuaig's *The Weariness, the Fever, and the Fret: The Campaign Against Tuberculosis in Canada* is excellent (McGill-Queen's University Press, 1995). Pat Sandiford Grygier's book, *A Long Way from Home: The Tuberculosis Epidemic Among the Inuit* (McGill-Queen's University Press, 1994), does something tellingly unusual in the history of TB books, which is talk about the disease from the patients' perspective.

In terms of local medical history, I found David B. Stewart's book *Holy Ground: The Story of the Manitoba Sanatorium at Ninette* enormously useful (J.A. Victor David Museum, 1999), as was Ian Carr's and Robert E. Beamish's book,

Manitoba Medicine: A Brief History (University of Manitoba Press, 1999). For the institutional history of the Sanatorium Board of Manitoba, I relied a great deal on the annual reports of the Board and of the Manitoba Lung Association. Sheppy Hershfield's memoirs were both important sources for this book: *Medical Memories* and *I Remember When* (both self-published, 1973 and ca. 1970). Joann MacMorran's reference book *Tuberculosis: A Handbook for Public Health Nurses and Other Health Care Workers* (Manitoba Department of Health, 1997, 3rd ed.) was very helpful to me in understanding TB control work here in Manitoba. John S. Milloy's book *A National Crime: The Canadian Government and the Residential School System, 1879-1986* was my primary reference for the history of residential schools in western Canada (University of Manitoba Press, 1999). For the early history of Winnipeg I drew especially on Alan Artibise's books, *Winnipeg: A Social History of Urban Growth 1874–1914* (McGill-Queen's University Press, Montreal and London, 1975), and *Gateway City: Documents on the City of Winnipeg 1873–1913* (the Manitoba Record Society and the University of Manitoba Press, 1979).

Among older books on TB the classic is still *The White Plague: Tuberculosis, Man, and Society,* by René and Jean Dubos, first published in 1952 (Rutgers University Press reprint, 1987). Dubos coined the phrase "think globally and act locally" in 1972, and the book he wrote on TB with his wife is every bit as relevant today as it was more than half a century ago. F.B. Smith's *The Retreat of Tuberculosis: 1850-1950* is elegantly written and packed with interesting details about the sanatorium era in particular (Croom Helm, 1988). Linda Bryder's book, *Below the Magic Mountain: A Social History of Tuberculosis in Twentieth-Century Britain* was also informative on the social history of sanatoria (Clarendon Press, 1988).

Frank Ryan's *The Forgotten Plague: How the Battle Against Tuberculosis Was Won – and Lost* is the best single source for reading about the lives of scientists whose work figures prominently in the history of TB (Little Brown and Company, 1992). Paul Farmer's book *Pathologies of Power: Health, Human Rights, and the New War on the Poor* is a good counterbalance to reading in the medical literature because it is so politically engaged (University of California Press, 2003). Tracy Kidder's book about Paul Farmer, *Mountains Beyond Mountains* (Random House, 2003) is inspirational and illuminating.

I found two books by American scholars useful for my purposes, Sheila M. Rothman's *Living in the Shadow of Deaths: Tuberculosis and the Social Experience of Illness in American History* (Johns Hopkins University Press, 1994), and *Disease and Class: Tuberculosis and the Shaping of Modern North American Society,* by Georgina D. Feldberg (Rutgers University Press, 1995).

Most of the current Canadian statistics on TB are available in full on the Internet. Health Canada publishes an annual report called "Tuberculosis in Canada." The most recent edition is for 2001. You can find it at

<www.hc-sc.gc.ca/pphb-dgspsp/publicat/tbcan01/index.html> (published 2003). Previous "Tuberculosis in Canada" annual reports from 1996 to 2000 can be found at <http://www.hc-sc.gc.ca/pphb-dgspsp/publications_2_e.html>. Also at this last URL you can find annual reports on TB drug resistance in Canada from 1998 to 2003. The "Canadian Tuberculosis Standards" (5th edition, 2000), to which Earl Hershfield was a contributor, are available at <www.hc-sc.gc.ca/pphb-dgspsp/tbpc-latb/pubs_e.html>.

Much of the recent statistical information on TB and Canadian Aboriginal people is publically accessible on-line. For a recent statistical overview of Aboriginal health, I used "A Statistical Profile on the Health of First Nations in Canada" (Health Canada, 2003), available at <www.hc-sc.gc.ca/fnihb-dgspni/fnihb/sppa/hia/publications/statistical_profile.htm>. More specialized information on TB can be found in "Special Report of the Canadian Tuberculosis Committee: Tuberculosis in Canadian-born Aboriginal Peoples" (Health Canada, 2002), at <http://www.hc-sc.gc.ca/pphb-dgspsp/publicat/tbcbap-tbpac/special_report_e.html>. I also drew on information in "Tuberculosis in First Nations Communities (Health Canada, 1999), at <www.hc-sc.gc.ca/fnihb/phcph/tuberculosis/publications/tuberculosis_fnc.pdf>, to which Earl Hershfield once again was a contributor.

For information on TB globally, I recommend the World Health Organization's web site, with a good starting point at <www.who.int/health_topics/tuberculosis/en/>. The WHO is also the definitive source of international health statistics. All the TB-focused international organizations I mention in the book can be easily found using the Google search engine.

INDEX